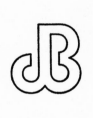

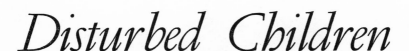

Disturbed Children

Examination and Assessment
Through Team Process

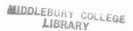

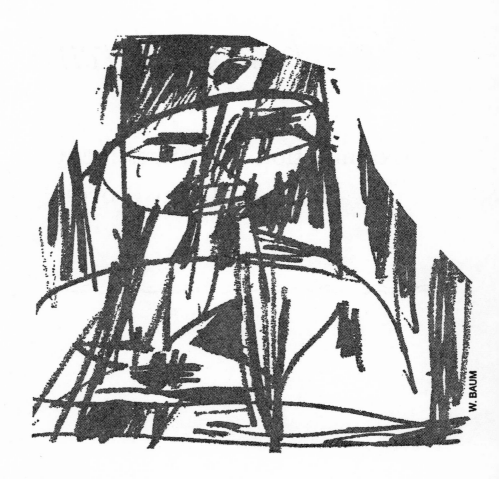

W. BAUM

disturbed children

By the Staff of the
Menninger Clinic Children's Division
The Menninger Foundation

Jossey-Bass Inc., Publishers
615 Montgomery Street • San Francisco • 1969

3/1970
Genl.

DISTURBED CHILDREN
Examination and Assessment through Team Process
by The Menninger Clinic Children's Division

Jossey-Bass, Inc., Publishers
615 Montgomery Street
San Francisco, California 94111

Library of Congress Catalog Card Number 68–54941

Standard Book Number SBN 87589–042–3

Manufactured in the United States of America
    Composed and printed by York Composition Company, Inc.
    Bound by Chas. H. Bohn & Co., Inc., New York
    Jacket design by Willi Baum, San Francisco

FIRST EDITION

Code 6910

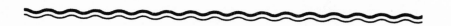

THE JOSSEY-BASS BEHAVIORAL SCIENCE SERIES

General Editors

WILLIAM E. HENRY, *University of Chicago*

NEVITT SANFORD, *Stanford University and Wright Institute, Berkeley*

To

    the patients, the parents,
the staff, and the setting
that made it possible

Preface

Elmer Ernest Southard was one of the great leaders in American psychiatry. "Go back to Kansas," he said to one of his students at Harvard Medical School, Karl Menninger, "and establish a psychiatric clinic; but don't forget the children! It is from them that we are going to learn most about the human mind and therefore about mental health." Through the inspiration of Dr. Southard's teaching, the Southard School came into being in 1926 as a partnership between the Menninger Sanitarium and a teacher, Miss Stella Pearson. In the beginning it was a small residential school whose program centered around the training of young children who were functioning at a retarded level. It was not long, however, before the school became fully a part of the Menninger Clinic; many changes of program over the years have brought the school to its current residential treatment program for disturbed children and youth. This evolution included housing at three different addresses in renovated old private residences but always with the dream of a permanent, planned new home to house the expanding treatment program. In 1961, that dream came true with the dedication of the Children's Hospital of the Menninger Clinic.

Another aspect of the evolution of child psychiatry at the Menninger Clinic was the development of outpatient diagnostic service. This clinical activity also underwent many changes during the time that child psychiatry and the related disciplines were coming of age.

In 1915, William Healy stated in his book, *The Individual Delinquent:* "The delinquent is the product of conditions and forces which have been actively forming him from the earliest moment of unicellular life. The facts of ancestry, antenatal life, child development, illnesses and injuries, social experiences and the vast field of mental life lead to invaluable understandings of the individual and to some idea of that wonderful complex of results which we term personality." While Healy was referring particularly to delinquents, our present understanding of psychiatric disturbances, made possible by psychoanalysis, emphasizes that all our diagnoses must consider and include a large variety of interlocking factors. These need to be identified and understood before therapeutic intervention can take place.

In this book we spell out how these many factors are elicited, elaborated, integrated, and utilized in the diagnostic work we do at the Menninger Clinic with the children who are brought to us for outpatient examinations. For us, the fact that our patients are growing and maturing individuals is a crucial factor which deserves careful attention. Delay, deviation, or disturbance in any one aspect of growth and maturation may impair, retard, or block a child's overall development, even though nature later compensates for it or the residual effects become less and less important as the child grows older. For example, a child's premature puberty at the age of eight may separate him from his peers by introducing new impulses and new psychological dilemmas at a time when he is too emotionally immature to deal with these problems. As he grows up the dilemmas may decrease, yet the child's psyche may have suffered serious harm in the meantime. Such psychological damage may, in turn, make it harder for him to meet the stresses of the adolescent years. In addition, children continue to be more or less dependent on their parents. We are striving to understand more and more about the effect that parents' conscious and unconscious conflicts and values have on their children's immature conscious and unconscious processes. We are also deeply interested in the extremely lively emotional interaction which takes place in families.

Parents who put little stress on intellectual performance may find it easier to accept apparent retardation in one of their children than parents who are college graduates with many intellectual interests. Such parents are liable to suffer a great deal as they see their child struggle to perform even simple intellectual tasks. Their conflicted feelings and attitudes are reflected back to the child and can be a large influence on how the child views himself and his capacities. The child may become very discouraged and preoccupied with methods that help him avoid displaying his lack of efficiency. As a result, he may find it harder to learn or to progress within the limits of his ability. Such slowness may aggravate the parents' reactions and thus the vicious circle goes. In such cases, a "diagnosis" made only by examining the child is not only insufficient but grossly inaccurate. A careful assessment of the child within the family must be included in order to reach a diagnostic understanding that will lead to recommendations relating to all of the etiologic factors responsible for his and his family's tension.

The psychiatric diagnosis of a child is an extremely complex process, which at the very minimum considers congenital, gestational, maturational, physiological, neurological, psychological, parental, familial, cultural, religious, and socioeconomic factors. We believe that no single professional discipline can hope to en-

compass or claim such a process exclusively as its own; consequently, child psychiatrists must avail themselves of the help offered
by colleagues in many other related disciplines. Several years ago,
Karl Menninger, addressing a large audience of internists, said,
"But we must have a diagnosis. Yes, but the question is: Who
is the 'we'? Do you mean 'we' internists? 'we' neurologists? 'we'
pathologists? 'we' sociologists? 'we' psychologists? 'we' psychiatrists?
All of us are interested in the same individual; we all believe in the
same scientific laws; we are all studying the same inter-related
phenomena. Yet each of us has his own little list of syndromes, and
we look for symptoms to fit the preconception without reference to
any other 'we' and call that a diagnosis. And just as surely as we do
that, we violate the basic principle of the modern holistic or totalis-
tic concept of the human organism. In theory there cannot be any
such thing as a simple uncomplicated diagnosis of anything, not
even measles. The child with the measles has at the same time some
educational interruptions, and some social complications, and some
disturbed relationships with parents and siblings."

Certain of the ideas contained in this book were formulated
during teaching sessions with fellows in the training program in
child psychiatry, with postdoctoral fellows in child psychology, and
with post-master's-degree trainees in social work at the Children's
Division of the Menninger Clinic. Support for these training programs has been graciously supplied by The Grant Foundation, The
Seeley Foundation, The Sloan Foundation, The Field Foundation,
and the National Institute of Mental Health. One of the primary
functions of the Menninger Clinic is to study, diagnose, and treat
the psychiatric problems not only of people living within our community but of those who come to us from a distance. In discharging
that function, we offer diagnostic and treatment services to parents
and children, as well as consultative services to public and private
agencies throughout the city of Topeka, the state of Kansas, and
to other places widely scattered over the nation. Such a balance of
diagnosis, treatment, teaching, and research and preventive functions has given dynamic and creative character to our work and
we hope to this book; we also hope that it will help others in their
efforts to relieve the suffering and to sustain the emotional strengths

of those children and parents who for various reasons have been unable to make full use of the resources that they possess.

Although we embrace the concept of prevention and early intervention, this book does not directly concern itself with what is now called "the new community psychiatry," which involves working in a community with the problems of many children by directing the efforts of many kinds of helpers and interviewers at many levels. For us that is another book. The basic body of knowledge of the various disciplines working with disturbed children comes from the records of one-to-one interactions between therapist and child and the study-in-depth of the family. After having mastered the basic skills acquired in this type of intensive experience, the individual and the team will be prepared to move into the community and modify those skills to meet widely varying situations.

Primarily, this book is about "the team," which, with the increasing understanding of its members, can play a more effective role in diagnosis. We present our concepts of the team and the team process. We say "team process" because we believe that the diagnostic study of a child is more than a series of isolated examinations and reports; it is more than the sum of the parts. The findings, the insights, and the conclusions of each individual on the team contribute to those of the other members as the examination proceeds; consequently, this process makes for a more carefully considered, integrated, and comprehensive diagnosis. The day-by-day sharing of the findings among the members of the team and the collective thinking of the team contribute to a greater understanding and acceptance of the diagnosis by the parents who have participated in each step of this process. The result is better treatment planning and recommendations which the parents are also more likely to support.

This book—which we have spent more than ten years in writing—gives a broad picture of the work as it goes on each week at The Menninger Foundation. Each professional approach is described by those who represent it, and integrative chapters show the operation as a whole. In the last several years two of the contributors have moved from the Foundation: Keith Bryant is now in private practice of child psychiatry and child psychoanalysis in La Jolla, California; and Povl Toussieng is now at the University of Oklahoma School of Medicine in Oklahoma City.

ACKNOWLEDGMENTS

Our indebtedness to Karl Menninger and Elmer Ernest Southard has already been mentioned. We are no less indebted to C. F. Menninger and William C. Menninger. We are also grateful to George Gardner of Boston, Roy Mendelsohn of St. Louis, and Reginald Lourie and his staff of Washington, D.C., for their critical reviews of the manuscript at various stages of the writing.

A complete list of acknowledgments would include many of the staff of The Menninger Foundation over the last decade. Two colleagues, Lois B. Murphy and Gardner Murphy, are to be thanked explicitly for the editorial skill and devotion they put into this writing effort. Our deepest thanks also go to Hazelle Bruce, Mary Jane Beatty, Rita Garrett, Marian Phelps, and Judy Walton for their guardianship of the changing manuscript over the years of writing and rewriting; to our librarian, Vesta Walker, who checked the bibliography; and to Lillabelle Stahl who helped with the final preparation of the material. We particularly wish to thank Virginia Eicholtz for preparing the index and for her careful editing and correcting of the proof. Lester Roach, executive secretary of The Menninger Foundation, along with Basil Cole, administrative assistant to the director of the Children's Division, must also be cited for their unwavering encouragement and support of this project.

August, 1969   ROBERT E. SWITZER
Topeka, Kansas   J. COTTER HIRSCHBERG

Contents

xvii

The Authors

Keith Bryant, M.D., psychiatrist

Ernest A. Hirsch, Ph.D., psychologist

J. Cotter Hirschberg, M.D., child psychoanalyst

Arthur Mandelbaum, M.S.W., chief psychiatric
social worker

J. Tarlton Morrow, Jr., M.D., training director

Lois Barclay Murphy, Ph.D., research psychologist

Clyde L. Rousey, Ph.D., speech pathologist

Joseph Stein, M.D., neurologist

Robert E. Switzer, M.D., director,
Children's Division

Disturbed Children

Examination and Assessment Through Team Process

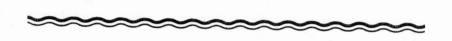

CHAPTER I

Diagnosis: A Team Process

A diagnostic study of a child by a psychiatrist usually takes a relatively short time and essentially provides only a view of the child's present functioning. The diagnostic findings, however, gain meaning the more they can be related to the past, in which the child's problem arose, to the vital present, and to the future, in which treatment of the child and other actions or changes in the living arrangement, schooling, and so forth—recommended as a result of the study—will be implemented. Since the main victims of the problem, the child and his parents, are also the very agents who will have to carry out the recommended treatment, the outlook for success depends on the depth of their commitment to follow the recommendations. This commitment will be greater in proportion to their genuine understanding of the nature of the problem and the factors contributing to it. The process of collecting as complete information as possible about the child's (and the family's) history and background will not only contribute added depth to the diagnostic study, it will engage the family in examining and understanding the history and origins of the problem. In this way they will begin to be active during the diagnostic study itself. The more the family and the child participate actively in the diagnostic process, with a sense of being respected and also understood, the more ready they will be to grasp, accept, and follow a treatment plan.

MOBILIZATION OF STRENGTH

If the child has very serious problems, he and his parents may feel utterly defeated. Then they will be likely to present themselves as specimens for diagnostic scrutiny under a microscope and they may expect to take no active role in the study. If the diagnostic examination is done on this basis, the family members will still feel helpless and defeated at the end of the study, and recommendations made to them then will only add to their burden further and to their existing feeling of hoplessness. Little action to implement or support treatment can be expected from them under such circumstances. However, if they have been able to participate more actively in the diagnostic process itself, they may acquire a beginning awareness of their potential strengths. They may draw increasingly on these strengths in the diagnostic process itself and this will greatly enhance the likelihood of their mobilizing psychological resources needed to sustain the treatment recommended. Despair will have been replaced by some hope and the likelihood of a successful outcome of treatment will be increased. This deepened involvement of the child and family in the diagnostic and treatment phases will also reduce their dependency on professional help after the examination.

Even in less severe cases, a deliberate and active mobilization of family members' strengths throughout the diagnostic process is likely to lead to their participating more confidently in the treatment which follows. Based on these considerations, the diagnostic studies described in this book have a twofold purpose: (1) to obtain as much information as possible on the child and his family and to use this information to reach a thorough understanding of the nature, scope, etiology, and development of the problem which caused the family to seek help; and (2) to use the data-gathering process itself as a device to involve the parents and the child in a thorough self-examination while exploring the problem. Knowing what to look for and why, parents can, with support, provide information which they might otherwise consider too trivial or too embarrassing to mention. Thus, the opportunity of the diagnostic team to reach a deeper understanding is enhanced.

While a great number of families coming to our clinic are self-referred, the majority are referred by their family physician, the child's therapist, a clinic, an agency, or some other professional source. Frequently, the person or clinic making the referral is also the first to make contact with us, sometimes with the offer to make all the necessary preparations with us for the study. For the reasons outlined above, however, we generally ask that the referral source request the parents themselves to write or call us directly. When they do this, the parents are involved from the start in an active process of seeking change. This request is particularly important because some parents tend to hide behind the referral source, out of embarrassment or anxiety. They may express dismay or even indignation when they themselves are asked to state the reason for seeking the diagnostic examination. Often reacting the same way are those self-referred parents who failed in their initial inquiry to give their child's age, name, and sex, the nature of his problem, and sometimes even the type of help they are seeking.

Tactful handling of parents' reactions and behavior over the phone or by correspondence may help them realize how defensive they have become about having a sick or difficult child, how anxious they are regarding this step they are about to take, and how difficult it is for them to admit or see that their child has a problem. The clinic staff member's respect for the parents' feelings, as well as his quiet expression of confidence that the parents can do what is necessary, helps them to mobilize their strength so they can begin to take an increasingly active role in preparing for the examination. At the same time, the clinic staff obtains valuable clues as to parental feelings, attitudes, expectations, and underlying motivations. Careful study of the correspondence and of other records from the parents will provide further clues and will enable the diagnostic team to start with the family at a much more informed level.

Valuable clues are also obtained from the parents' reactions to the requirements that (1) both of them should be available for daily interviews throughout the examinations; (2) both should write out a history of the child's life and send it to the clinic in advance; (3) they should send pictures of the child showing him at various ages from birth to present time; and (4) they should get in touch with all the professional people who in any capacity have had contact with the child and authorize them to send us a report of their impressions and findings. These reports should include letters from the child's teachers, as well as from the family physician or pediatrician. For those parents who complain that they were never involved in any important way in any examination of, or work with, their child, never given anything to do, never made to feel useful during the examination, the above requests initiate a personal involvement, which is likely to deepen after the study begins. Such parents experience their efforts as important from the start, and frequently view the preparations as evidence of the clinic's thoroughness and eagerness to know the child fully. Other parents, however, react to the clinic's requests with varying degrees of discomfort or anxiety. They may be frightened that their child will appear extremely ill, or not as ill as they believe he is; or they may be so disappointed, frightened, or angry about past examinations that they may not even wish, for example, to have the upcoming study influenced, or contaminated, by previous reports from examiners. If properly understood, these parents' struggles can also be utilized to engage both mother and father actively in the examination process before the actual study of the child has started at the clinic.

> *Case Example:* A staff member made a phone call to the mother of a child scheduled for examination to inform her that reports from three psychiatrists, two of whom were psychoanalysts, had not been received. The mother promptly became argumentative and angry. She told a lengthy story about the incredible "psychoanalytic mess" existing in the large metropolitan center where she lives and called the doctors who were to send the reports "absolute frauds." These people had conspired against her and her husband, she said. For this reason she and her husband had decided they would not let the doctors write reports to us, since they wanted us to give them our unbiased opinion. If we got these reports, we would be set against the parents. If they left Topeka having some doubts about the outcome of the examination, they would always continue to think that the reports we had received from the previous psychiatrist had influenced us. She repeated that she had not gotten any help whatsoever from these people, and actually they had made it more difficult to get help for her son.
>
> We promptly explained to the mother what her refusal of this information implied. For one thing, it meant she had doubts about our professional integrity even before meeting us. What effect would this have on the outcome of the examination? How readily would she and her husband believe what we had to say under these circumstances? The mother became more angry, complaining that she was being "psychoanalyzed" over the phone. She stressed that she and her husband had discussed not sending the medical reports. They were in unanimous agreement about this, and they wanted it done their way. We stressed in reply that the question was not merely whether

or not we would get the reports, as we were more concerned about the reason for the parents' refusal to cooperate. Our staff very much wanted to help them but it
seemed now that the family would arrive here with a
"closed fist," as it were, rather than with an open hand.
As a result, they might go away angry and disappointed
and feel cheated.

The mother calmed down a little bit, saying that
she knew she had strong and angry feelings but that she
and her husband had been "squelched" earlier by doctors.
We accepted her fears and told her we could understand
how they could influence her attitude toward the clinic.
At this point, she began to stress how meaningful our
letters had been, how different they were from the previous
professional contacts she had experienced. She said that
though she and her husband were placing restrictions on
our staff, they felt this action would have value for the
future, even though they would come away from the clinic
feeling somewhat let down. She said that the other doctors
had always told them that their resistance stood in the
way of helping their son; if we independently came up
with the same opinion, they would know that they had
been wrong in their view of their son's problems. We
pointed out that they seemed to expect to be on trial here.
Yet, so far all our contacts with them, including this one,
had reflected their genuine wish to help their son. The
issue as to whether the parents had shown resistance,
therefore, really was irrelevant at the present time; the
only issue was to figure out how the son could best be
helped. With this, there was a dramatic shift in the
mother's voice, which became so very quiet, that she sometimes was almost inaudible. She stated that this call really
had raised some important issues and promised that she
and her husband would think it through again.

It is clear from this conversation that strong feelings prevented the parents from using their previous professional contacts

constructively and that the pain caused by what they had been told had proved unbearable. They had reacted to the pain by becoming angry, hurt, and defensive because they experienced the medical conclusions as attacks on their parental integrity and their worth as parents. Even so, their continuing awareness of their child's problems and suffering compelled them once again to make an attempt to seek help. Whether or not they will have the reports forwarded after the above phone call is much less important than their having already recognized before the start of the study that they genuinely desire to help their child, and that this very wish causes them anxiety. Thus, when they arrive for their first appointment, their attitude and focus will be different from those they would have if they had not been asked to take the responsibility for having the professional reports sent.

These reports are of great value to the diagnostic team, and the primary purpose of data gathering before the study begins is not to test for or produce reactions in the parents. Such a deception would be absurd and cruel, designed merely to keep the parents busy instead of involved out of real need. Nor is the purpose of data gathering to give the appearance of thoroughness because of volume. Rather, facts are a vital necessity for understanding the child in earlier stages of development, and through this understanding to have a sounder view of the factors in his present functioning, and also a more adequate evaluation of his potentialities, as well as his present needs for help.

The request for the parents to write out a history and be present throughout the examination does not mean they will participate primarily as informants. Their participation helps them to clarify not only the sequences in the child's development but their own attitudes toward and feelings about the child and his problems. A child's difficulties affect and have roots in the total family. Therefore, the participation of the child and his parents in the entire diagnostic process provides current examples of family interactions and emotional responses; as the family members themselves begin to look at these interactions, they become more receptive to a thorough assessment of the problem and to a plan for effective therapy.

Even if one parent gives compelling reasons for not accompanying the child to the diagnostic study, it still is essential not
to accept these excuses immediately but to discuss them as part of
the initial exploration with the parents. Almost invariably the
reasons given appear less prohibitive when discussed in the light
of the parents' expressed wish to make the most of the diagnostic
study and to seek effective help for their child. Rarely after such
clarification does a parent not proceed with the plan for the study
once he has convinced himself that the clinic really believes his
participation to be essential. Thus, parents who cooperate fully
express at the same time their willingness to work on changing
what they had earlier thought was impossible to change. The busy
physician father who "could not possibly be away from his practice
that long" finds a way to come anyway because he finds he is more
deeply concerned about his child than his practice. A mother who
cannot come because she is recuperating from a serious illness decides that she "has more strength than she realized." The father
who has a new job and cannot yet ask for a vacation nevertheless
finds he is concerned enough about his child to speak to his em-
ployer. He not only gets the necessary leave but sometimes an offer
from his company to underwrite part of the examination expenses.
The divorced mother who has custody of the child and wants no
contact with her former husband finally gets in touch with him
and is surprised by his concern—a concern that is encouraged because his wife's call shows him he is an important figure in the
child's life in spite of the marital breakdown. In all these instances,
the resolving of the complexities of participation represent an explicit recognition both of the compelling and serious nature of the
child's problem and the parents' deep solicitude. It also reflects
hope and faith that something can be done after all and that the
parents think they have the strength to cope with the problem.

However, should one parent continue to refuse to come or
insist he cannot come, the clarification process still is essential.
There is the question as to how adequately the parent who does
come can convey to the other parent what findings and recommendations have resulted from this study. Significant family tensions

and struggles can remain hidden during the study if the parent most involved in these difficulties is absent.

Parents from the local area are not dealt with by phone or letters alone but are always invited to come in together for an intake interview with a psychiatric social worker. These interviews are structured on the basis of the same philosophy and viewpoint mentioned above (see Chapter Two). At times a child psychiatrist also sees the child in consultation in order to determine whether a more comprehensive study is desirable. The circumstances surrounding the actual diagnostic study of the child can also be of great help in the total process. The fact that both parents have taken time out to participate in a study, with all the accompanying demands this effort makes in terms of travel, expense, and special arrangements, can have an intense meaning to the child who has many doubts about his parents' love for him; sometimes it can be used as a takeoff point in the child's interviews with the psychiatrist. The special attention the child receives during the study may make it possible for him to relax, to cooperate better, and to function at his optimum level. The parents' conviction about the study also conveys their willingness and determination to change things in the family as a whole and in the child in particular.

> *Case Example:* After an examination date for his fourteen-year-old son had already been set, the father called to check whether all the reports on the boy had been received. He then asked whether it would be okay not to tell his son about the examination until they were on their way to the first appointment Monday morning. The staff member asked him why he would want to handle the situation this way, and he immediately insisted that otherwise there would be no way of getting the boy to Topeka. The son would refuse to come. An empathic discussion of the father's helplessness followed with the firm request that he tell his son before leaving for Topeka. The father's anxiety regarding this request was recognized and discussed as evidence of the magnitude of the problem with

which the parents were struggling. The staff member also stressed to the father that an examination, of course, would be impossible if the boy was not physically available for his appointments. Someone would also need to be willing to support the boy in coming for his interviews when and if the child did not have the strength to take the responsibility for this himself. The father agreed, stating that something had to be done and promising that he would tell the boy in advance. He added that he personally would see to it that the boy was at the clinic Monday morning.

While living in close quarters at a hotel or motel with the child or while spending much time with him between appointments, family members can rarely maintain an attitude of aloofness or deny the existence of their problem. During the study itself the feeling of "bursting with emotion" (Modlin, Gardner, and Faris, 1958) produced in family members by their interviews, as well as by their internal pressures toward change and greater psychological health, also pushes them toward more meaningful communication with each other. Sometimes this communication is on a level on which they have not talked for a long time, or maybe never before. In these heart-to-heart talks, husband and wife, parents and child may face reality together for the first time, often with intense relief in spite of the anxiety they may feel (and with which the diagnostic team will have to deal). The fact that all three family members are away from the drudgeries and pressures of their work and life at home further enhances this diagnostic process, because of the fewer escape hatches and the greater opportunity to focus exclusively on the problem at hand. Many fathers, after experiencing their children's exhausting behavioral problems at the hotel or in the waiting room, have exclaimed that they were unaware of what their wives were going through and were sorry that they had not done something about the situation sooner.

If the diagnostic process is successful the family members will be better prepared to bear up under the findings and recommendations at the end of the study and it will be more difficult for them to remain aloof from the professional opinions. We may, therefore, sum up the above considerations by again emphasizing our conviction that all contacts with the family from the very start should be used not only in the overall diagnostic process but also to help the family members move toward greater self-awareness and a wider perspective in relation to the child's difficulties, so they can mobilize and use their strengths to make the necessary changes.

TEAM PROCESS

The child guidance movement early recognized the multiple factors which had to be considered when dealing with children. As a result it drew upon the membership in the fields of psychiatry, psychology, and social work in setting up psychiatric teams. At the Children's Division of the Menninger Clinic this team consists not only of members from these three professions but also from neurology, neuropsychology, and sometimes from various other disciplines, such as speech and hearing pathology, internal medicine, pediatrics. This diversity is considered necessary particularly because of the complexity of the problems brought to our clinic. More than half the children examined over the years in Topeka come from distant places. In the ten years from July 1, 1957, to July 1, 1967, the Children's Division examined 655 children. Of this number, 269 were from the Kansas area; 386 came from other states. As excellent diagnostic and therapeutic psychiatric facilities for children are becoming increasingly available throughout most of the United States, children and their parents are not referred for examination here, so far away from home, unless major differential-diagnostic difficulties exist or unless all local helping resources have been exhausted. Consequently—particularly compared with the usual children's psychiatric clinic—a disproportionately large percentage of children with serious problems is examined here (see Table 1).

It is against this background that the diagnostic procedures that are used at the Menninger Clinic must be understood. The reader will consistently need to keep this in mind as we describe our techniques and procedures. Furthermore, the Children's Division is part of a private institution; thus compared with most children's

Table 1

Distribution of Primary Diagnoses

(451 males, 204 females)

Disturbances associated with organic processes[a]	177
Mental deficiency[b]	26
Behavior disorders of childhood[c]	57
Character disorders[c]	87
Psychoneurotic reactions[c]	158
Psychotic reactions[c]	147
Psychiatric disease, none	3
Total:	655

[a] Some of these children were also found to be emotionally disturbed or retarded, but the primary difficulty was believed to be the organic impairment.

[b] Listed are only those children in whom mental deficiency was the primary and only diagnosis.

[c] Some of these children also showed some organic impairment or mental deficiency.

psychiatric clinics, our center sees a larger percentage of families from the middle or upper-middle class. It is necessary then to emphasize that this book is not written to spell out how the authors think *all* psychiatric examinations of children should be done. We merely want to share our diagnostic methods and thinking, in the hope that colleagues in other clinics will review them and find them useful to compare with their own diagnostic philosophy and methods.

Our diagnostic procedures not only reflect our approach to doing an examination but also our way of viewing psychiatric diagnosis, or our philosophy as to how such a diagnosis can best be reached. For us the comprehensive understanding of a difficult problem in a child makes "diagnosis" such a complex concept that no one professional discipline can completely encompass it. In these difficult cases, as we have mentioned before, we always arrange for people from a number of professional disciplines to participate in the study and use their skills in the overall diagnostic effort. However, if these various people did not work together as a team, but merely communicated their findings to each other, their efforts would fail to have the unity essential to the clinic's high standards for diagnosis. However, before such professionals as a psychiatrist, a psychiatric social worker, a psychologist, a neurologist, and a speech and hearing pathologist can become a psychiatric team capable of making a thorough diagnosis, they must learn to work closely together and understand each other's professional terms and philosophy. Their communication cannot remain confined to the formal conferences alone but must extend to include such informal ways as phone calls and casual conversation. These casual discussions help to clarify confusing or conflicting points which have emerged in the examinations. In this way, each team member not only struggles to understand or formulate clearly the diagnostic information he obtains through his own professional tools but also participates completely in the team effort to put all these pieces of information together as the diagnosis reflects a thoroughly integrated understanding of the child's and the family's total situation. We discuss this process in Chapters Eight and Nine.

Genetic, biologic, historical, and laboratory data must all be integrated with the impressions gained in psychiatric interviews with the child, as well as with the results from the psychological tests. The child's physical and neurological status, his defenses, impulses, needs, conflicts, assets and liabilities, psychosexual maturity, and object relationships must be assessed. The psychological aspects of the child's functioning are explored by determining how he behaves, how he interacts with and is viewed in his usual environment, both at home and elsewhere. Much of this information is obtained from the casework with the parents. The parents' attitudes and feelings toward the child need to be identified and understood, in the light of their own background, education, religion, and socioeconomic status. All of these data must eventually be weighed in order to understand whether the child's psychological growth and maturation have become blocked; if so, exactly how, and what effects these blocks have had on the child, his parents, and sometimes, as well, on the community at large.

Like other clinics, we have to fit this information under a diagnostic label, which, at best, is only a faint indication of the overall diagnostic understanding and cannot be made to include every piece of crucial and significant data. The label *school phobia,* for example, tells us nothing as to the child's intellectual potential or as to how the mother may unconsciously trigger and aggravate his problem. Nor does the label *mental retardation* tell us that perhaps the child's ambitious, professional parents cannot keep from pushing him toward a performance level which he cannot possibly reach, with the result that his self-esteem is severely damaged from his failure to please his parents. Labels are useful in professional communication, but they lose their value when their use only supports diagnosis as a static concept. As conceptualized here, diagnosis is a dynamic, and inclusive, concept, which begins—but does not end—with the examination.

Regardless of the label attached to a child's disturbance, attention must be given equally to the tensions in his family and to the question of whether or not these tensions originate in the child's problem. Where there is a disturbed child there usually is a disturbed family, and the original source of the problem may well reside some place other than where the family places it at the time of referral. The psychiatric team can easily be led astray by the initial complaint and then fail to give due weight to other factors. If a mother "needs" the child's disturbance so she can devote all her time to him and thus have a good excuse for withdrawing from her husband, any treatment offered the child will remain ineffective until the adult difficulties have been brought out in the open and worked through or alleviated. Factors in the larger environment in which the family lives may also play a vital role in a child's or family's disturbance. Evaluating these factors can pose many difficulties. Because families come from far away, we often cannot quite assess such things as the local subculture, religious traditions, and socioeconomic tensions, but, nevertheless, we make every effort to clarify this aspect of the diagnostic picture, too.

The problems of how to set up a team and how to help it function at its best are discussed in Chapter Nine. We need only stress here that each member must learn to use himself in a way that will also enhance the work of others on the team. For example, he might seek additional information that will clarify the ambiguous or incomplete findings of another team member. In one instance, a psychologist obtained from a child many stories with themes of violence on the Thematic Apperception Test. He then gave this information to the social worker, who had told him that the parents had denied, so far, the presence of any kind of marital discord. Aided by this knowledge, the social worker helped the parents to share the knowledge of, and their guilts about, marital battles fought out in front of the child. In another instance, the neurologist on a team reported suspicion of increased intracranial pressure in a child who was being examined for a severe school phobia—a child who vomited every time an attempt was made to get him to go to school. Up to this point the dynamics of the situation had been the classical ones of a school phobia with severe conflicts in the child regarding the mother and with a history of lifelong phobia in the mother. Nevertheless, the neurological findings on this child, as well as certain evidence in the psychological tests, clearly indicated that he was suffering from a brain tumor rather than from a school phobia. In another case, the team psychologist told the psychiatrist that the child with whom they were working seemed deeply burdened by something. With this in mind the latter, through skillful exploration, learned about the mother's serious alcoholism, which the family so far had kept a closely guarded secret.

This last example brings up the point that the family members also have a collaborative role in the overall diagnostic effort. They, too, must "participate actively in the solution of the clinical problem which they originally brought (Modlin, Gardner, and Faris, 1958)." This does not mean, of course, that the family members will be expected to help identify certain neurological disorders or help score psychological tests, but it does mean that they must constantly be made aware of what information (which only they can contribute) will be relevant and that they, too, must help weigh the relative importance of this material. If they can assume this role, their understanding of themselves and each other will inevitably deepen and will change their position in relation to the problem. In this way they become readier to help formulate and accept an appropriate and workable treatment plan—usually the most important goal of a diagnostic study.

The change that takes place in the family members can be viewed as a therapeutic effect of the examination process and is an important one because it does not come about merely by doing a study. The professional team members assume that family members will give in proportion to what they feel they are receiving during the study. The more support, understanding, and clarification the team can offer them, the freer the family members will feel to "open up" and to contribute information which otherwise would remain hidden, because they consider it too dangerous, too frightening, or too painful to reveal.

When the family arrives, the disturbed interaction patterns between individual family members, as well as the family's wishes and expectations, are often projected onto the clinic setting and the team. The parents of a retarded child, for example, may project a feeling that the team's findings must be completely negative or that a complete cure must be possible. A team aware of these projections avoids stepping into the role assigned by the family and instead uses such projected wishes to clarify with the parents the many fears, doubts, and angers underlying these hopes. It will then be possible to explore with them what is realistically possible and what is impossible. The team then acts as a support and a mirror to the family and sets the stage so that the individual members, by actively participating themselves, can gain new insights into their difficulties.

PROCEDURAL STRUCTURE

In preparing the reader for the chapters to follow, we must now turn to the actual structure and procedures of our psychiatric examinations. Here, as in any clinic, the structure of the examination is determined not only by purely psychiatric goals but also by administrative, financial, geographic, and other considerations. For example, the examination structure must be sufficiently flexible to adjust to the varying demands presented by the cases from outside Topeka, which are usually very difficult and complex, and the local cases, which are generally common enough to be seen in any child guidance clinic. In order to limit the expense of the examination and not to make the family's absence from home so long that it becomes disruptive, the study has been set to take five to six days. It starts on a Monday morning and ends on a Friday evening, or even occasionally on Saturday morning.

Compressing a comprehensive diagnostic study into a five-day period is a major problem and makes great demands on the family's ability to cooperate. This applies particularly to the child, who may have as many as four or five appointments in one day. The five-day period may, in fact, be barely long enough to get through to the child, particularly if he has difficulty in making new contacts or in tolerating interpersonal situations, if he fatigues easily, or is excessively afraid or angry. He and his parents can move and change only so much in that short a time span, and sometimes major psychological resistances simply cannot be worked through in the period. The professional team is therefore under heavy pressure, as it must reach some level of dynamic understanding of the child's and the parents' defenses, character patterns, attitudes, and emotional difficulties, in order to find a way to support the family emotionally and to map a strategy as to how each member can best be freed to participate meaningfully in the examination.

Before the family arrives, the team gets together for an hour with the senior staff psychiatrist who will be the team consultant for this study and will chair all the conferences. In this conference the available reports and other information are reviewed, and examination procedures are planned. The decision may be made, for instance, whether the social worker and the psychiatrist should have a joint session with the entire family before the doctor takes the child to his office. Additional laboratory procedures or special psychological tests not usually used in examinations may also be decided upon at this time. If other relatives accompany the family— they sometimes do, particularly if one parent is dead—plans are made as to whether the social worker will also talk with them and if so, to what extent.

When the family members come in for their first appointment on Monday morning, they are met by the person on the staff with whom they corresponded; he introduces them to the social worker, who will see the parents, and to the child psychiatrist, who will see the child. The parents are usually seen together in the first interview, but subsequently the social worker structures daily individual or joint interviews with them on a flexible basis, determined by the needs of the case. The psychiatrist sees the child daily for one hour and uses part of one of these sessions to do a psychiatric physical examination, as described by Levy (1929). Later Monday morning, the psychiatrist introduces the child to the psychologist, who sees the child at least twice daily until all testing goals have been accomplished. On the second or third day, the child is examined by the neurologist, who first takes the medical history in an interview with both parents. As his office is much closer to the laboratory, the neurologist is also the one who shows the child the laboratory, explains the EEG machine (electroencephalograph), and answers any questions the youngster may have.

All children have X-rays of the skull, the chest, and the wrists (for "bone-age"—a rough, but fast, appraisal of hormonal functioning), an EEG (wake, sleep, hyperventilation, and photic stimulation), blood tests (CBC, differential count, mean corpuscular hemoglobin, hematocrit, VDRL, blood type, and Rh factor), and urine studies (specific gravity, gross appearance, pH, microscopy, albumin, sugar, and four metabolic screening tests: phenylpyruvic acid, DNPH, Benedict's, and nitroprusside). Additional laboratory work is ordered if indicated. All of these studies are usually done the day after the neurological examination.

The speech and hearing specialist sees all children routinely. However, the neurophysiologist, the pediatrician, and other medical specialists see the children only on special referral. Interviews with these team members are worked into the schedule as appointments can be obtained, but are scheduled during the last half of the study if possible, as the child is more likely to be cooperative and relaxed by then.

On Wednesday afternoon, most children have a testing session with the psychologist in a one-way vision room. Here the psychiatrist and the social worker also have an opportunity to observe the child through the mirror, and other staff members frequently sit in, providing a further occasion for observation and consultation.

The reason for having so many of these examination procedures and tests so regularly deserves further discussion. As already mentioned, many of these procedures and tests are usually necessary to settle the complex differential-diagnostic questions brought to us.

However, beyond this factor we are impressed with the need to study carefully each child's physical and neurological status, as there are significant findings in this area in at least half of the children studied here—even in the children from the local area (see Chapter Six). The fact that a child is underweight or undersized, is late going into puberty, or has congenital stigmata or an abnormal EEG may not in itself have major significance, but it may still contribute vitally not only to the overall understanding of the child and his difficulties but to the final diagnosis as well. For example, the diagnosis of congenital aphasia sometimes can be considered as a possibility only on the basis of many cues, each insignificant in itself but suggestive as a group. Many frustrating years may be lost in trying to help the child through psychotherapy alone if the diagnosis of aphasia is missed. In spite of the cost and the many additional hours required, we therefore continue to see our team procedures as an irreducible minimum.

Early Wednesday morning, at the so-called preconference, the team members share in a more systematic way their findings and observations with each other and the consultant. A tentative formulation of the case is made and the recommendations which possibly may come out of the examination are discussed, so that the social worker and the psychiatrist can begin to explore the parents' and the child's feelings as to future action. Friday afternoon from 1:00 to 3:00 P.M., all the team members and the consultant get together for a final conference. The team members bring in prepared reports and the final diagnosis synthesis, from which they will formulate a treatment plan. Prepared reports, rather than informal presentations, are considered to be important because they force team members to sift, digest, and integrate their observations and to state them in a clear, organized, and coherent fashion. From 3:00 to 5:00 P.M., the psychiatrist joins the social worker and the parents to discuss the findings, while the more extensive discussion of the recommendations usually is conducted by the social worker alone after the doctor has left. If the child is old enough—and whenever there is an indication for it—the psychiatrist also talks to the child about the outcome of the study and the treatment recommendations. However, great flexibility is exercised in these arrangements, so that the psychiatrist, for example, may remain with the parents and the social worker to discuss the recommendations, or the psychiatrist and the child may join the parents and the social worker after they have talked alone first. The social worker and the psychiatrist are available to the family for further interviews on Saturday morning if further discussion is necessary.

Much care goes into the writing of reports to the professional people who referred the family or who will be working with the family to implement the recommendations. This is a difficult task, and it must be given proper emphasis. However well the diagnostic study was done, findings and recommendations may be useless if they are not conveyed to colleagues in such a way that they can understand and thus continue with the family the process started here at Topeka. At the clinic a guide has been devised for organizing professional observations in a purposeful and coherent way (K. Menninger, 1962). Even so, written reports continue to be a major challenge.

Our team members are keenly aware of the difficulties inherent in diagnostic work and in conveying their professional observations and conclusions to the family and professional colleagues. The ideal goal in every evaluation is elusive, and errors in judgment or understanding most certainly occur. For the sake of future patients, as well as for the purpose of further staff development, we try to review all errors. If an examination does not end satisfactorily, an understanding of the causes for the difficulty will gradually increase staff members' ability to accomplish better team efficiency and collaboration, thus enhancing their ability to work more usefully with difficult families and problems. Even so, a number of cases remain where our knowledge, experience, and skills are still insufficient to deal with the problems presented by certain children and their parents within the total socioeconomic and cultural context. A dedicated staff, driven by a healthy and constructive concern, continues to search for new ways of handling these difficulties. This book is one step in our search for answers to the problems with which we, and many of our colleagues across the land, have to grapple far too often.

CHAPTER II

Working with Parents

The parents of a physically or emotionally ill child must make the important decision as to when outside help is required. In most instances, they have the adult power to take action, some knowledge of treatment resources—however rudimentary—and the financial ability to pay for help. They may act quickly when the child's symptoms become acute or painful and they feel helpless to relieve his distress. In the case of physical illness, the symptoms at least are relatively tangible and clear, and the physician, although he may be viewed with some apprehension, is, nevertheless, a familiar figure who they believe will know what to do. Eager to carry out his directions, the parents feel useful, important, and needed, even if they are only asked to give a pill, take a temperature, or sit by their child's bedside.

But emotional illness in a child is a mysterious and frightening thing, because the child cannot point to any particular place where his body hurts. He cannot define the specific nature of his distress but must express it through symptoms which often seem irrational and without cause. The parents are sometimes solaced by thinking that these symptoms are a temporary manifestation, like previous plateaus of growth and development, and thus will disappear on their own. That there may be an actual distortion or halting of development is indeed a difficult judgment for them to make. One parent may reassure the other; usually the mother is reassured by the father, who is less likely to see the child's behavior throughout most of the day. He will point to the positive and gratifying achievements of the child.

Nor can the child help very much to dispel this false reassurance. He may not even know that he is ill, that his behavior is strange and differs in degree from that of the other children. He may have only the vaguest sense of discomfort, unhappiness, and irritability, and no understanding of why he cries without apparent cause. His dilemma, however, does not result in psychiatric help unless its impact involves and is felt by the parents. When they are drawn into the child's distress, when they sense his pain as, in part, indistinguishable from their own and are bewildered and angry when their own attempts at giving help fail, they may seek outside assistance. Before they reach this point, though, they have felt pain, frustration, and confusion. They have had frantic, searching inner thoughts concerning their possible contributions to the child's problem. Often they view the child's illness as an aggressive act designed to hurt and control them—a willful, bad act which the child could master if he chose to do so. They may even feel that the child wishes to humiliate them.

Case Example: Charles, age twelve, ran away from home the day after receiving his first report card on which he had flunked every subject. (As Mrs. B. talked, her story became somewhat confused, so that her husband gently interrupted and took over.) Charles, despite considerable pressure, stubbornly refuses to apply himself to his lessons unless his father is willing to study with him every night. He has run away from home three or four times. The last time, he stole several guns, one of which was from a neighbor, and then stole some money and stayed out all night. The children in the neighborhood now call him a thief, and all the teachers know of his difficulties. The parents feel Charles is worse than ever before, since he is nasty and mean to his brother and talks back to his mother. His mother is frightened of him. Although he has no difficulty going to school, often he will phone his mother to come for him after school is out, giving her the excuse that the other children are waiting to beat him. Both parents feel that Charles in some way feels he deserves being beaten by others and, therefore, makes no effort to fight back. This is in contrast to his increased quarreling with Donald, who is ten years old and the only other sibling. There is also increased nastiness to his mother. The parents described Charles as sulking and angry when at home, refusing to do anything around the house or becoming enthusiastic about some activity only to abandon it before completing the project. Both parents were at a loss to describe Charles and his interests except in contrast to his younger brother, Donald, who is gay, competent, and a good student. Donald does everything to please them; Charles only frightens and angers them. They are always after him to make an effort to do well.

WHY PARENTS COME

It is never easy for parents to make up their minds to bring a child for a psychiatric examination. There is none of the quality of, "It's about time we take him to the dentist for a checkup." The decision to inquire about psychiatric help is always the outcome, to some degree, of a crisis in the family. This crisis threatens the accustomed equilibrium of family life in such a way as to cause deep discomfort in the relationship between the parents, their individual relationships to the child, and to the other offspring in the family. In this sense, it is family crisis; the tension exists among its members and is confined to the home, or else spills out into the community. It does not usually originate in the community. The family crisis may reach the point where the parents threaten each other with abandonment and want help with this threat to family unity. They may define the problem in terms of the child because they sense he threatens their psychic stability and their control over their anger. With some guilt, parents may express the wish to know the effect of family tensions on the child, but underlying this is the fear of what such tensions mean about their adequacies. They may suspect that it is they who need psychiatric help but come to get help for the child since he is the focal point of disturbance; he absorbs and reflects the conflicts in themselves.

Case Example: Mrs. A. spoke of how upset she is and the fact that her husband now threatens to separate from the family. She said that he can go if he wishes to do so. She would keep custody of the child and would insist on this. She does not care about living with her husband any longer and has no feeling for him other than disgust. The worker commented that she seemed shocked to learn of her husband's intentions. Mrs. A. agreed, and there were tears in her eyes as she spoke of being abandoned and rejected at this critical time when they were trying to help the child. She attacked her husband's inadequacy, his excessive dependency on her, his resentment and criticism of the care she gives the child, his anger when the house is upset and untidy, his accusation that she is not a good mother, and his failure to realize the enormous difficulties the child presents to her and to everyone. She wondered whether the worker saw the justification of her position and whether he thought her right.

The parents may also come for help because they fear loss of control over the child; in other words, his behavior is becoming too powerful to control and confine only to the home situation. There is fear about the future or of deep-rooted disturbances in themselves which go back to their own childhood.

Pressure for help may come, however, from a combination of internal and external sources. It is rare that the child confines his disturbed behavior to the home situation alone. It is also rare that reasons for coming for help are based on one or two factors; rather, they involve a multiplicity of interacting elements. The pediatrician, for example, may sense something is wrong when he cannot find a physical basis for somatic complaints and suspects that frequent school absences are due to an emotional problem which underlies physical symptoms. The school, now increasingly more alert and sensitive to children who do not perform well, may quickly call the parents' attention to the child who cannot learn, concentrate, or relax in the classroom. Neighbors, the police, and the juvenile court are also far less hesitant to involve parents when their child causes disruptive behavior in the community. These external signs that something is wrong reflect the internal anxieties and struggles of the family, and they combine to place heightened pressure on the parents to seek a course of constructive action.

Case Example: Mrs. C., a forty-year-old widow, lost her husband several years ago when he committed suicide. He had been despondent for many years, and she had had to rescue him from many business failures and law suits. Her daughter, Sally, an only child, seemed shadowy and insubstantial to both the father, when he was alive, and to Mrs. C., who had had to give so much attention to her husband. Sally, now fifteen, had done fairly well in school during the elementary grades, but she had been a quiet, withdrawn, and lonely child. In high school, her academic work began to decline; as she observed her mother's increasing depression and drinking, she began to stay away from home, finally running off with another girl to a distant city, where the police found her living in a motel. Her

behavior seemed to be like a cry of distress expressed both
for herself and her mother, finally forcing Mrs. C. to
apply for help.

The major conception of the diagnostic study is that as
understanding of the total nature of the patient's problems and the
problems of family interaction increases, a plan of action gradually
emerges designed to help the patient and his family resolve their
difficulties. The diagnostic study is the preparation for treatment.
The worker proceeds in this direction by having the parents take a
long, intense look at the problems they bring and the goals they
seek. Parents examine the quality of relationships they have with
the patient, as well as his personality and behavior difficulties, and
out of the increased clarity which emerges, since they are less hampered by anger and fear, they will know better what to do. The
parents and the worker have a sense that there is an end point to
the process, a summing up, when all they have thought about, felt,
and understood as well as they could, will lead to making choices—
perhaps difficult and frustrating choices—so that the best design
for treatment can evolve. As they work hard together, they have an
awareness of the limits of time and an awareness that they must all
consider what the parents want to do and are able to do, framed
further by the realities of what help this setting or other resources
can give. These are the natural limits of the study, dictated by a
host of factors which, through careful deliberation, the worker can
regard as essential or relevant, or can ignore or bypass for other
solutions.

There must be action within the study—action that causes
the parents to join with the worker in the task of sorting material
and illuminating important ideas and feelings. As parents sort
material, they will discard some data as relatively unimportant and
will bring other data to the forefront to assume a proper place in
the scheme of things or rearrange to make coherent and understandable what was obscure or chaotic before. This systematizing
and conscious recognition of the complexities of the problem gradually become related to what the other team members are doing;

as a result, their combined understanding of the totality will lead to a concept of what should and can be done for the patient and his family.

As the worker accumulates a series of impressions of what the parents are like and what their relationship is like with the patient, he accumulates impressions at the same time of how the parents view themselves and their interaction with their child. He also gets a view of the parents as they react to him, as well as their view of this interaction. He must, in the end, put all of these impressions together, so that he can see them all at once and as a whole, just as they are in real life, and thus simultaneously see their varied, shifting changes and complexities. If you also add the impressions of the child obtained concurrently by the psychiatrists and the psychologists, who aim, too, for this kind of total view, then you get an understanding of the illness as it actually pervades the environment and all relationships in that environment.

The skill of the worker is manifested in the way he sets in motion and guides this exploration, making full use of the meaning of the material so that the capacity of the parents to deal with it is constantly strengthened. The worker controls the process of change in the direction of what goals must be considered as a result of what is being learned in the study. At the end of the study, the parents should have arrived at a new intellectual and emotional understanding of their troubled life experiences with their child—an understanding which will now make their interaction together more significant and more fruitful.

Within this general conception of a process in which the psychiatric social worker and parents struggle together to understand the problem, certain questions are especially important to answer. We have discussed above the question of why parents come for help. But only during the exploration does the further question of why they come at a particular time get a clear answer. Under the disorganizing pressures of anxiety and torn by indecision, most parents need ample time to describe in their own ways what has impelled them to seek help now and at this agency. It is not unusual for parents who have sought help elsewhere to complain about the insufficient time and attention they were given. They frequently point out that their story was only half heard and understood, their child was seen too briefly, and that the recommendations, which they comprehended only vaguely, appeared to have been based on snap judgments and hasty distortions caused by their anger and anxiety. In this way the social worker gains some sense of the parents' manner and style of dealing with intense feelings.

Many times, the parents themselves do not know why specifically they come for help at this time. They are dimly aware, if at all, of causes and precipitating events. They are not even sure they can convey something they themselves but faintly understand, and, most important of all, they are not sure that their own gropings to understand the true source of their distress will be met with kindness, sufficient time, and sufficient care. Great stress produces feelings of isolation, loneliness, and heightened anxiety. Under such tensions, thought and reflection are submerged by the rush of impulse and action toward quick sedation; what the sedation is does not matter as long as it relieves immediate pain. Since some of the behavior of the parents and child prior to coming for help seemed to be purposeless and chaotic, the beginning procedures are designed to give the parents sufficient pause so that anxiety and impulses to action can be turned into thought, reflection, and then the wisest choice of action possible.

The question as to whether the child himself needs help, and if so, what kind, is not easily answered. Only after the early anxieties of the parents are allayed can the examination explore the patient's need for help and the ways to proceed. The parents ask for help but their readiness to use the kind of service the clinic has to offer may vary from genuine bewilderment as to whether there are difficulties requiring outside professional assistance to an expressed sincere belief that their child has a serious problem and requires psychiatric treatment. The task of evaluating the real need for help is complicated by the ambivalence of some parents: their overt reluctance and distaste for any self-involvement, and their vague description of difficulties reflect their resistance. The parents may minimize the problem and give a description of it designed to shield its seriousness from themselves as well as from the interviewer. The task is easier when parents describe the problem in dramatic terms to underscore that they must be believed and they want relief and change.

> *Case Example:* After the first incident of their child's running away from home, Mr. and Mrs. T. consulted with the psychiatrist who gave consultation to the public school system. They were concerned at that time that Timothy was not doing well in school and was possibly upset. They felt they needed help in knowing how to handle him. Dr. A. gave them the impression that they had handled the entire situation in the worst possible manner and that Timothy was a very insecure child and felt himself unwanted and unloved. This was quite disturbing to the parents and they have since tried to handle Timothy with kid gloves, not punishing him for his recent escapade and, in fact, relieving all pressure on him insofar as school work is concerned. They feel that Timothy is worse than ever now.
>
> Before Mrs. T. talked to Dr. A., she was able to handle Timothy spontaneously and intuitively; now she ponders and broods over her reactions, sometimes becoming too paralyzed to say or do anything with him.

Fear of Involvement

Parents usually come at a time of intense crisis, at a "critical moment of living (Perlman, 1960, p. 171)." Their indecisiveness is at a high pitch and they are moving along a path of many divisions, some which go toward constructive solutions, and others toward a continuance of angry action to no purpose except that it gives themselves and others the guise of attempting a solution. Above all, the parents want relief for the child and for themselves. They wish to be understood and hope the interviewer will be their ally. They fear judgment and criticism, and their sensitivity to these reactions is raw and keen, a state of mind typical for all who are under heavy stress.

Although parents lend themselves to an inquiry and exploration of their problems with their child, they are concerned about the wisdom of doing so. In the case example above, the parents felt attacked; moreover, they had experienced the psychiatrist as an intruder who had rendered them not more but less effective than before. Whether this was actually so might be debated, but it is not the heart of the matter. Regardless of the accuracy of their belief, this is their perception of what happened and how they were affected. Therefore, the core issue is their expectation of a similar experience here and their determination perhaps to see it this way. This perception of the current process is sure to be colored by the past and interferes with the attempt to perceive it as it is now.

Parents' fears become a vital subject for discussion and one of the important themes in the psychiatric study. It is not surprising that the parents are so fearful of criticism. Their child's illness is, in effect, a tacit accusation that they have not been able to meet his needs. From every direction, including their own inner thoughts, they are subject to critical comment. Emotional illness is still considered a social stigma but, even more, it means that parents have failed in human relationships in a culture and society which take failure hard and reject it as intolerable.

This fear of blame is one of the reasons why parents go many other places before they come to the psychiatric clinic. They also fear what they may be told, fear they will be ridiculed and humiliated, fear that their rage and anger will be exposed and become openly explosive and destructive, fear that their feelings of inadequacy will be increased. In this strange and unfamiliar place, they are not quite sure what will be required of them or how much of themselves, their own thoughts, and their views and opinions of their difficulties will be involved. They fear the normal pattern of their lives may be altered by a professional person who, initially symbolizing a critical and authoritative figure, may demand changes of an unpleasant nature, will intrude and investigate, and may even take parental controls away from them. All of these fears clash against the wishes for help and set up a defensive struggle, as illustrated in the following case.

Case Example: Mr. and Mrs. S. were referred by their pediatrician because their three-year-old son, Leonard, was having frightening dreams, which began at the extremely early age of two-and-one-half months. The parents described him as afraid of being separated from his mother; he objected and cried when they planned to go out in the evening. Mrs. S. is a tall, attractive woman who gazed at the worker intently as if trying to judge his thoughts about her. She spoke rapidly and under great pressure. When the worker reflected her fears of coming, she agreed and spoke of the criticisms made of her by her in-laws.

Leonard will fall asleep only fitfully throughout the night until his mother consents to sleep with him. He says he is frightened of shadows and pictures on the wall, and he seems "to be actually seeing things not there." Leonard was raised on a strict schedule and to avoid his crying after a certain period of time, Mrs. S. would overfeed him and he would throw up. She criticized her doctors for not helping with this problem, for being critical of her overfeeding the infant, and rather pathetically she stated, "Leonard can work me." Mrs. S. said she then began to sleep with Leonard in order to calm him. Her husband became angry and would spank the child. Although she has tried to separate from him throughout the night, it has not worked. She described her own childhood as consisting of a series of difficult separations from key figures, especially her mother. "I lacked affection," she said.

Mr. S. thought Leonard was a fearful, headstrong, stubborn child whose eyes were "for his mother and very seldom for me." He thought they had spoiled the boy and had been too lenient with him. He appeared concerned that he would have to participate in an evaluation. His schedule would not permit this, he said. Mrs. S. was disappointed that immediate advice might not handle the situation, and she spoke of Leonard's fears of tornadoes and storms as if to equate these with psychiatric help.

She felt that she and her husband would not have the strength to ride through such storms.

Beginning Participation

In discussing preparation for child analysis, Anna Freud (1946) made the point that "insight into the seriousness of the neurosis, the decision to begin and to continue treatment, persistence in the face of resistance or of passing aggravations of the illness, are beyond the child and have to be supplied by the parents. In child analysis, the parents' good sense plays the part which the healthy part of the patient's conscious personality plays during adult analysis to safeguard and maintain the continuance of treatment (p. 69)."

The beginning of the process is designed to free the parents' good sense in favor of the child. But, in such a beginning, each parent is given the opportunity to present his individual concerns and the depth of his personal reactions about his emotional investment.

Few couples view the child's problems in the same way, and it is not surprising that they seldom are united in their struggle to find a solution. An important function of the initial interviews is to help the parents resolve at least one part of their conflicting views: namely, are they able to reach agreement that what the child needs is of paramount importance to him and to themselves? If they can agree in this one area, some of their competitiveness and inconsistency yields to their recognition that both they and their child can use help.

The very act of coming to the clinic means that, at least tentatively, the parents have agreed to talk about their problems. This decision brings with it many defenses, but as the worker responds to the parents—listening with concentrated attention to their story, and observing the interaction between them and with him— this activity takes direction from a host of factors flowing toward him in a swift stream.

He observes carefully the actions and the physical and emotional aspects of each parent, such as the timbre of their voices, the expression of their eyes and facial features, their posture, their choice of where they sit (whether near or far from him and each other), the removal of their coats or insistence upon remaining wrapped in them. Their attitudes toward each other and to him show the areas where there is agreement or conflict.

He permits free expression of feeling, observing how spontaneous the parents are about speaking in each other's presence. If he senses excessive inhibition and fear between the parents, he will swiftly decide in his own mind as to the value of separate, rather than joint, interviews throughout the diagnostic study.

He observes how closely the parents concentrate on the child's problems or whether they are more concerned with their own individual need for help, or help with their marital relationship.

He will raise questions about the relationship between parents and child, accepting the fact as valid that they are not using the child as a screen or as an excuse for their own need for help but are genuinely disturbed about the child's problems. He will maintain this focus unless it becomes clear to him and the parents that their concentration on themselves is a defensive device due to their fright about their child or that they genuinely want help for themselves.

He takes seriously the parents' fright and apprehension and comments upon it warmly and appropriately. His questions and requests for clarification are expressed so that the parents soon recognize that because much is unclear to him, much is also unclear to them. Thus, the worker's activity is designed to enlarge mutual understanding.

In turn, he does not assume that the parents understand the clinic, its purpose, procedures, and its special language and particular expertness. He will explain clearly and simply to the parents in what ways the clinic may be able to help with their problem, what they can expect from such help, the time and costs involved, what other things will be expected of them, and what they can require from the clinic. The fact that the parents have decided to come is never accepted at face value to mean that they have no ambivalence about coming; as a result, the process consistently assists the parents to explore their doubts and clarify their own thoughts as to what they want and what will be involved.

He is aware of the parents' fears at the outset and, therefore, their sensitivity to any threatening attitudes of his such as dislike, contempt, subtle blame or his identification with the child against them—any or all of which may serve to justify their decision not to use the recommendations which will emerge from the study.

Although one of the goals of the worker is to accumulate knowledge about the child and his problems and the core nature of his relationship with his parents, the worker's central purpose is to use this knowledge in such a way that the parents will accept the final recommendations. This was assisted when during the study they found it a relief to express their feelings, doubts, and fears. In other words, their intense concerns were met with respect and understanding, the expected criticism and punishment were not forthcoming, and they learned a number of invaluable facts about themselves as well as about their child. They learned that they could talk and that they were not alone in having fears, since the worker did not seem to view them as unique or strange. The clear, skillful way he asked and organized questions gave the promise that they might learn about their child something that would be useful to the task of living with him. It is this sense of being treated with respect and dignity, of learning something, and of having the hope of learning even more that engages the parents and leads to the decision to make as effective use of the recommendations as possible.

First Family Contact

When the family—with whom the clinic had no previous personal contact except through phone calls and correspondence— arrives from out of town, all participants in the study, including the diagnostic team, feel some measure of anxiety. The family members' basic purpose is to protect, maintain, and enhance their self-concept. They wish to show their strengths, as well as their anxieties and deep concerns. In turn, the members of the professional team wish to bring to the task their finest skills. They also wish to maintain and enhance their own self-esteem. The difference between the family and the professional team is that the family comes with feelings of failure and is already trying to fend off a poor self-concept and poor self-esteem. Overwhelmed with anxiety, the family may first show its more regressive aspects, and if team participants are not alert to this possibility, they will overestimate the family's weaknesses and pathology and not see the potential strength that can flourish under their careful use of skill and warmth. The child deals with the double burden of his parents' sadness and anger toward him and his own self-doubts and anger. Any beginning process must take these important emotions into account and safeguard against deepening them.

The process must be structured so that each member of the family can give his view of the misfortunes that have befallen him; in addition, it should help him to pull himself together to work on his problems and show his strengths as well as his emotional difficulties. The question for the team is how best to begin such a process. Perhaps valuable cues may be obtained not only from a clear conception of the purpose of family interviewing but also from a careful examination of all the material that comes to the clinic prior to the family's arrival. The first contact may be a joint procedure involving the parents, child, social worker, and psychiatrist; or the child can immediately separate from his parents and see the psychiatrist alone, while his parents are interviewed by the social worker.

The joint interview provides the opportunity to have each member of the family engage in an interaction which, although it takes place under stress and with strangers involved, nevertheless gives a clear idea of what strong as well as subtle nuances of feeling are present. Each individual has a chance to present his view of the problem, why he thinks the family has come, why they have a problem, and what help they want or do not want. In the presence of neutral observers, each has the opportunity to learn how together or apart they are in their views, how conflicting and competitive, how clashing and discordant. What further emerges is how truthful the parents have been with the child about his coming; have they been frank and courageous enough to share with him their belief that he and they have a problem in living together and have now come for help? Or it may emerge that they are so fearful of the child, so much controlled by his irrational behavior, that they are unable, both from anger and fear, to confront him with the realities of his difficulties. Despite the careful preparations by the outpatient director, who has corresponded with the family, the parents may not have been able to tell the child where he is going and the reason why.

In the joint interview, each individual gives some clue as to the characteristic defense position he will use. Both parents may project the fault onto a series of external circumstances which have always placed the child and themselves at the constant disadvantage of being embattled against the world. One or both may threaten the child with the psychiatric study as punishment or as a way of discovering who is the guilty party causing family difficulty. The father may insist that the mother is the person responsible, or the mother may use the situation to berate her husband for his neglect, unfaithfulness, or failure to invest himself emotionally. Both parents may criticize the child and unite to expose him for his behavior, or the child may attack both of his parents and accuse them of being too punitive, too strict, or perhaps too overly permissive. Thus, each individual may react in the way best affording protection for the safety of his self-esteem and self-regard.

The social worker and psychiatrist have multiple functions in the joint interview. Both are introduced to the family simultaneously, so the parents and the child have the opportunity to meet together the individuals with whom they will work most intensely. Both wish to encourage the parents and the child to express themselves freely and to experience the social worker and the psychiatrist as committed to empathy with the family; they are not allied with any one person against the others. Both social worker and psychiatrist act as weights in the joint interview, giving it balance so that all individuals get a chance to be heard; no one person is permitted to dominate or to lacerate others so that they feel unduly exposed and unfairly attacked without a chance to counterbalance and neutralize such aggression.

The clinicians have the opportunity to observe and experience the emotional climate created by the family, the ways they relate and use each other, and the choice and use of words which

reveal the communication methods of this family group. Not un-
expectedly, each family member senses himself in danger, in danger
of exposure and of being blamed, in danger of losing control over
painful feelings, and in danger of saying the wrong things. But, in
addition, he feels a relief in being heard, of having a chance to talk
in a structured situation where it is also possible to be understood;
surrounded by numbers, he has, as well, the chance to observe and
hear in safety the complaints and grievances of other members of
the family, who may earlier have been too timid to express themselves or who, feeling both the pressure and the protection of the
group, may reveal things only half felt, half perceived, or even mis-
understood before.

The joint interview has immediate therapeutic elements,
which manifest themselves through the acceptance of what each
member has to say: the respectful attention, dignity, and intensity
of listening the team participants give to the family, their nonjudg-
mental attitudes; and their careful, discriminating comments and
behavior, which assist in facilitating the flow of feelings. Further,
the activity of the team has a specific focus in the beginning of the
process. The aim is not only to determine what each family member thinks the problem is, why they have come, and what they hope
to receive, but also to give back to each member a clear statement
of the purpose of the study, of how our clinic hopes to help, and
of the family's place and participation in the process. The parents
know then that they have an important place and responsibility in
the study; the patient knows that his needs, wishes, and hopes will
be given the most careful consideration and that he will have a
voice in decisions concerning his destiny. The joint interview can
then be a supportive experience for the whole family, with no private agreements or secret alliances. Since the destructive effects of
projection, competition, or wishes to escape can be discussed, these
can then be limited.

Because much of the diagnostic study of the child takes
place apart from the parents—in the psychiatrist's office and elsewhere—the joint interview provides the parents with a substantial
look at the psychiatrist who will be a major power in this process.
It also provides the child with a first impression of the doctor and

with the purpose of the social worker's activity. The social worker and psychiatrist, in turn, are given a chance to compare notes on the family in respect to the interaction they have observed, the feelings each individual has aroused in them, and the factors present or absent that seem to explain the patient's illness within this family. Thus, both psychiatrist and social worker start together and, although they then separate to pursue their goals in separate interviews, they have begun a process of weaving together what hitherto has been separate. At the end of the study, the entire team hopes to emerge with one fabric, placed and stitched together by members from the separate parts they have contributed.

Still another essential value of the joint process is that it gives the family the introductory experience of working together in a new way; here each is required, within a protected and structured situation, to explore and give some thought as to why they are having problems in living together. The interdependence of family members is emphasized; the interlocking nature of the problem is discussed; and it is made clear that any treatment plan proposed will acknowledge this interdependence and utilize its strengths to support the patient through negative as well as positive changes and through the ups and downs of treatment.

Sometimes, however, the joint interview may not be advisable. When the parents are overwhelmingly bitter and caustic with each other, a joint hour may serve no useful purpose and would, indeed, be only another frightening event to the child. If one or both parents are severely emotionally disturbed and disorganized and lack the ability to control thoughts and impulses, they are likely to find the swift interaction of a joint interview bewildering and frightening. However, even under these circumstances, skilled team members may, perhaps, lead the parents and child through a joint interview with benefit to all; but the hazards are sometimes complex and difficult to predict and control.

Since the value of a joint interview rests on all members being able to interact in at least some constructive capacity, those children who are inarticulate, severely retarded, or severely withdrawn cannot participate and exchange their thoughts and ideas. It may be argued that they are still participants even though on a primitive, infantile level. However, in such instances they are unable to state a point of view or to share their thoughts and thus cannot make the necessary changes for adjustment; their presence simply permits observation of their behavior in the group situation.

Occasionally, a child is so extremely hostile and suspicious of his parents and all other adults that he trusts no one. In such instances the child may decide not to communicate, not to utter a word that may endanger him; thus, by bitter silence he keeps control and power over the family. If he cannot control them by this method, he may choose to run.

> *Case Example:* When Mr. and Mrs. B. and their daughter, Nancy, age thirteen, were introduced to Dr. Vance and myself, the caseworker, they seated themselves opposite their child. Nancy sat in her chair with her arms folded hard and her legs held tightly together. Her eyes flashed angrily at her parents and her lips alternately clenched white and then opened wide, but no sounds emerged except an angry exhaling. I made a general comment as to their anxiety and tenseness about being here. The parents nodded. I went on to say that I knew the three of them had talked together about coming this week and it would be helpful to know what understanding they had about the reasons for coming. There was an immediate silence. The doctor commented that this was a difficult question for them. Mr. B. stated that one of the reasons concerned Nancy's academic work, that she wanted to go to a different high school, and didn't know where she could go or what courses she could study until she had taken some tests. Mrs. B. began to talk about Nancy's not doing well in school and her unhappiness over it. Nancy then spoke up and said she hated her name and her mother knew this. Dr. Vance wondered what Nancy liked to be called and she then said inaudibly, "Nelly."
>
> I attempted to redirect my question as to what difficulties had brought them here, other than school problems, mentioning that they had used the word *unhappy.*

I wondered whether Nancy was unhappy. At this point, Nancy looked at me in an angry way and stated that she had to go to the bathroom. As she left hurriedly, her mother called out to her that she must come right back. Nancy angrily replied that she would not come back until she felt like it. Dr. Vance then suggested that he go out and wait for her and they would then go to his office. I then spoke to the parents of Nancy's upsetting them and their fear of what she would do.

The psychiatrist's and social worker's observation of family interaction at the joint interview not only enhances the chance of an early integration of diagnostic thinking and planning but also permits them to test the confidence and respect they have for each other. The psychiatrist must be convinced that the social worker will say or do nothing to antagonize the child and thus make the process more difficult on that score. The social worker must be confident that the psychiatrist will do nothing to antagonize the parents and that he will create the proper climate in which everyone can participate to his maximum ability. Both must have the capacity to give their empathy to the whole family, rather than to a single individual; both must have a clear conception of the joint hour, what they hope it to accomplish, how far to allow aggression to be expressed, what areas to touch on, when to draw one particular individual further into the action and thus neutralize the activity of another, and when to signal the end of the interview as the beginning phase of the study.

HISTORY OF ILLNESS

In a sense, the history of the illness begins to be gathered at the very moment the parents inquire about help. In his interviews with the parents the social worker adds to this after the family arrives at the clinic. He is interested in the parents giving this history in any way they choose, selecting their own pace and their own style; at the same time, he comments on the uncomfortableness, fearfulness, and blocking that cause irrelevancies, undue detail, or vagueness—all of which add little understanding to the child's dilemma. The worker must repeatedly ask himself, "What anxieties cause these defenses and how can I reduce them?" if he is to get the most accurate, deeply felt, and deeply remembered picture of the patient's development and present illness.

The worker does not proceed by the question-and-answer method, for this is likely to produce sterile, matter-of-fact, and clipped answers; if he should proceed in this way, the parents would get the impression that his interest is simply in an organized, chronological, time-saving gathering of the material and not in their feelings or ideas as to what is wrong and the reasons for it. On the other hand, lack of guidance as to what the worker deems important or no increased interest or encouragement to talk when the parents are discussing an important point may leave them bewildered; or they may feel guilty about his sparing them a painful discussion of crucial events. The worker, then, must steer a careful course between too rigid guidance and no guidance of the interview. He indicates his interest in what the parents are saying by an encouraging nod, a simple yes, or by leaning forward to show a quickening of interest about some significant event. He does not press the parents to talk about events which seem excruciatingly painful but marks these areas as one places a buoy on the sea; he can navigate a return when the relationship is stronger and reflects more confidence. The worker's judgment regarding areas for further or more intensive exploration is based on his comprehensive knowledge of normal as well as pathological human growth and development, and life events which impede or enhance that development.

While slowly accumulating the data the worker is aware of what material will be of use to the psychologist, the psychiatrist, the neurologist, and the speech pathologist, all of whom will be seeing the child and his parents. He will organize the data into a picture of the child, his problem and its development, as given by the parents. He will supply the team with his appraisal of the problem, the clues he understands as important and worthy of further clarification. Of course, he will not present the material to the team as he received it, for in the give-and-take of interviews there are many side roads and blind alleys, as well as vital areas that are suddenly revealed and further exposed only to be covered again. A literal presentation would often be so disorganized that the other team members would be left with the task of giving coherence and meaning to the mass of material.

An outline for summarizing the case study is helpful. This one is taken from Karl Menninger's (1962) "Outline for Summarizing the Case Study" and is modified to make it useful to the work with parents.

I. Administrative data
  A. Name or file number, age, sex, nationality, ethnic group, marital status, occupation, religious affiliation, and place of normal residence. Names of father and mother, names and ages of siblings.
  B. Referring physician or agency.
  C. Administrative status of patient at the time of this summary.
II. Clinical data
  A. Historical data
    1. The "chief complaint" as given by referral sources; those contained in previous psychiatric examinations, or reports from the family physician, pediatrician, or juvenile court, leading to the initiation of the psychiatric case study.
    2. The background of the patient's life. This should begin with a brief description of the personality and background of the parents, particularly highlighting those events in the parents' backgrounds which might influence or which explain the patient's illness. A brief description of the motivations and events leading to the parents' marriage and events leading to the patient's birth. Economic, religious, cultural social status of the family before and after the patient's birth.
    Important events in the history of the family having to do with any unusual separations, illnesses or deaths, or any other traumatic events or persistent stress which might have had their influence on the child, his parents, and siblings.
    The birth history considers the physical and mental

health of the mother before and after delivery, parental attitudes about the addition of the particular child to the family, its sex, attractiveness. The infant history will cover the early adjustment reactions to life: feeding, sleeping, motor activities, reactions to cuddling, smiling, weaning, sitting up, walking and talking, bowel and bladder training, unusual illnesses, traumatic events. It will also cover those symptoms of infancy which concerned the parents such as thumbsucking, crying, fears, tics, masturbation, temper tantrums, and other behavior problems.

For some children, where deviations from normal development seem to be rooted in the very early developmental years, it may be necessary for the worker to gather data of a more detailed nature. Such an inventory might include items such as: vigor, expressiveness and ability to communicate needs, responsiveness and "sending power," irritability, sensitivity and reactivity to stimulation, including areas of hypersensitivity; activity level; ease of settling into a schedule; adaptability to change, newness, strangers; the capacity to tolerate delay, frustration, and separation. The parental attitudes toward these developmental items are of particular importance, giving clues to those nuances of feeling tone which suffused relationships between mother, father, the infant, his siblings, and other aspects of his environment.

Early childhood reactions to siblings, eating, teething, and sleeping patterns, separation anxieties and the adjustment to nursery school, if the child attends, and his relationships with peers. The sexual attitudes of the patient, and the ways in which the parents influence and respond to these.

If the patient is an adolescent, the history will take into account further data regarding his physical, mental and emotional development: his ability to emancipate from his parents, trends in sexual identification,

attitudes of the parents toward sexual patterns, play
and work habits in school and after school, evidences
of expectations and thought about the future, the
existence of neurotic symptoms or other ways the child
deals with anxieties, aggressive thoughts and feelings
and the parental attitudes toward the child's growing
up and their expectations of him.

III. Diagnostic and prognostic conclusions

    A. Appraisal of the parents

       The worker sums up his diagnostic impressions of the
parents; their assets and liabilities, their reactions to the
process, the growth or lack of growth in their understanding of themselves and the child, a summary of their
personality problems and difficulties especially as they
relate to the patient's illness and an estimate of the motivations and conflictual forces with which the parents
approached the study, and the ways they will likely deal
with the findings.

    B. Prognosis

      1. Accessibility of the parents to participation (motiva-
tion, cooperation, economics).

      2. Possibilities of changing the environment in a favor-
able direction.

FIRST HOUR WITH PARENTS

The first hour between the parents and social worker may
to some degree recapitulate the consultation process, if one was conducted with them. However, if the parents were not seen earlier in
consultation, they may repeat much of what they submitted in
writing as the history of their child's illness. Indeed, many parents
wearily detail the past, complaining that they have already told
the same story in many places. The worker must not be deceived
into believing that a repetition of the problem is stale, flat, and unprofitable. He is not, in fact, even hearing a replica of the consultation interview or of previous psychiatric contacts with the
family, for this is a new time and, in all probability, it is being told
to a new person and certainly under new, or at least different, cir-

cumstances. One important circumstance is that the parents are now committed to this venture, the decision to come is behind them, and a beginning has been made. Yet the parents probably have the same doubts they had in the psychiatric consultation sessions or with previous helping resources; thus, the worker must not take for granted that the parents have stopped doubting simply because they are now started in the diagnostic study. These doubts and misgivings will appear and reappear in many guises, some familiar and unfamiliar, as varied and rich in expression as the range of creativity in the individual parents. Each family must be viewed afresh, as a mystery or an enigma that challenges the worker's imagination and tests his perception and sensitivity.

The worker seeks to record the family's impact upon him, the quality and force of his experience with them. Simultaneously, the quality of his help comes from the effect of his warmth and understanding, which persuades the parents to open up to this new experience. In this intricate situation insights are generated for the parents and the team, insights which give the finest understanding of the child and his family.

The worker must go behind a facade, or a defense, to what is most frightening to the parents and persuade them to examine with him why they feel as they do about the patient and what they feel is tragic about their situation. It is not the worker who is unrelenting in this search but the parents' own torment that is unceasing. The worker tries to sense the nature of this torment, to imagine what it must feel like to them to experience it and then come with it to ask for help. If he can capture the parents' feeling, his attitude will give them a sense of their personal worth and dignity; and they will feel a lessening of their own apprehension concerning criticism, loss of self-esteem, and failure, because they do not find it in the worker.

This is the tone the worker strikes from the very beginning as he listens to the parents tell their story. As they accompany him to his office, everything they now say, do, and feel and everything he thinks, feels, and reacts to take a place within a frame where a picture is beginning to form. How the parents prepared the child for coming and how they separate from him, seemingly superficial chatter about their trip, whether it was difficult or easy, whether comfortable or tedious, tell a great deal of how they feel about being at the clinic. Even comments about the weather and their impressions of the physical surroundings give insight as to their feelings about the experience.

> *Case Example:* As the parents came with me, they wondered how long Ann would be with the doctor. Mrs. R. commented that Ann had gone willingly, had made no protest about seeing Dr. A. They began to explain while we were climbing the stairs that they had not told her that she was coming to see a psychiatrist. She was under the impression she was coming to see a doctor for physical evaluation; that the whole family was here for this purpose. By this time, we were in my office. Both commented on the steepness of the second stairway; it had taken their breath away. They commented also on the cold weather; they had not come prepared with winter clothing, so they were wearing two and three sweaters. They stated that this was an old building but we seemed to make adequate use of it and it was very well built. They had told Ann that she was coming for a medical checkup, not because they feared she would not come; she is a good sport, obedient, but they were afraid she would indiscriminately tell this to her friends and to others in the neighborhood. Their friends do not understand their seeking help for Ann; they are not aware of her problems, and they have not confided in them. After coming, Mr. R. told Ann how famous Hollywood movie stars were in treatment, and so this is a desirable place to come. They wanted her, he added, to feel happy and positive toward it.

The first hour is one in which themes are sounded that will reverberate throughout the study. The worker carefully sorts out these themes into those that are clearly recognizable by the parents, or only dimly perceived by them, or are far removed from their awareness. The techniques utilized include support and encouragement to speak thoughts and feelings, to explore ideas, to search memory, and to elaborate on casually or only vaguely mentioned details that might contain significant issues. Ambiguities, muddled thoughts, innuendoes, and suspicions are gently called to the attention of the parents, and they are asked to explain or enrich the content with feelings about it and whatever meaningful associations occur to the parents. When such techniques are used unobtrusively and with sensitivity as to how much intense exploration the parents can bear, they come to recognize the probing as a means of enlarging their understanding as well as the worker's and that both are interacting forces. The parents come to sense that, as the worker's understanding increases, their understanding broadens as well. Thus, the worker involves the parents in the service of the study, calling on their available strengths and maturity and relating to them as parents whose area of concern may include themselves as well as their child.

Foremost, the worker's activities deal with those emerging themes that are clearly most recognizable to the parents themselves. As they discuss their problem, it is relatively easy to comment on their concern about separation from the child in this current situation, their concern as to the status and nature of the people their child will be seeing, their views as to their reactions about being here, whom they are seeing, and attitudes toward previous professional people consulted. But the worker does not reflect these concerns until they are revealed, until they emerge. It is the parents who must take the lead, who must give the cues that this is what they are communicating. All too often the worker assumes that since many parents have certain feelings, all parents must have them, and that these feelings can be commented on in all situations because they must be there. This approach stereotypes individuals and makes interviews stilted and scattered; as a result, the parents may regard the worker as insensitive and rigid—an investigator seeking to discover "the crime."

Because the worker is familiar with psychological material and patterns of behavior and is accustomed to assigning meanings according to this knowledge, he may fail to question and to clarify material given by the parents, assuming that their intent is clear from what they are saying. When inferences, then, are based on inferences, the worker's foundation for understanding a family is indeed shaky.

In the security of his warm, comfortable office, where he knows the arrangement of the furniture, the color of the walls, and the warm, comforting books in his bookcase, the worker may be easily lulled into a sense of complacency, feeling that the parents are, or should be, as comfortable and secure as he is himself. To the parents, however, everything in the beginning is unfamiliar, strange, and cold. Recognition of this fact lessens the distance between them and the worker and begins with their most immediate feelings. Such an awareness follows the basic rule that it is wise to proceed from the familiar, from the known into less known areas. This procedure is most effective in proceeding cautiously to broader and deeper levels of understanding of family and problems.

The first hour, then, is a review of what is known, offering leads into what is less known. Under the pressure of anxiety and of being in a strange place, away from home, the parents produce a panorama of family difficulties in high relief, with the worker listening intently to their description of what is most discernible so they may eventually proceed together to less familiar territory. The circumstance of their coming, why they come now, what they see as the problem, and how and what they expect from help are beginnings. Feelings about the schedule, relief that it seems so thorough and so comprehensive, or fear of it, are also "beginning" feelings.

The fee for the diagnostic study should be reviewed in order to clarify the parents' understanding of it. As they consider what the study will cost them, fresh doubts and uncertainties will arise, and the parents may ask questions designed to obtain guarantees that the child will be cured; they may even wonder whether the study itself is the treatment and nothing further will be required. The worker can give no assurance of a cure. He can only promise that the team will attempt to understand the child as completely as possible, so that the clinic and the parents together will know the best treatment program to follow in the future. The worker will also emphasize that the study is not the treatment but a necessary preface to it. He may have to help the parents understand their wish for swift, absolute remedies without excessive cost, time, and the painful search into the past and present. The parents may then express fresh anger and insist that the child has not only emotionally exhausted them but will now deprive them of financial means. They may cite how this cost will deprive the other siblings and themselves of important necessities. The worker will recognize these protests about the fee as a reflection of the parents' underlying fears; these protests may also reflect unreadiness to proceed in the study, and fear of self-involvement. Unlike other services which are purchased—those requiring nothing from the buyer except the fee—the agreement to pay for psychiatric help involves more than money. It means an agreement to give freely of thoughts, ideas, and feelings and to subject these to self-examination with the help of another person. This is a dismaying fact to some parents. They are fearful because so much depends on them and because so much interest and attention will be focused on what they have to say. The payment of an agreed-upon fee will not absolve them of this responsibility.

The worker carries on the discussion about fees with the confidence and conviction that the clinic has a professional service which is worthy and highly valued. He reflects the scope and importance of the clinical procedures by his careful survey with the parents as to what they can realistically afford, not only for this present need but for what may be needed in the future. In this specific sense, the way the worker conducts the discussion of money has therapeutic value. His attempts to help the parents clarify what the fee means to them in relation to seeking help demonstrates that money has multiple meanings. An understanding of these meanings is part of the clinic's help.

Fees may sometimes be used to test the integrity of the setting and of the worker as a representative of that setting. One of the major problems with which parents struggle is that of trust. Since they have come to distrust and question their relationship to the child and fear the incendiary nature of their feelings much of this distrust and fear may be projected onto the clinic. Can they trust comparative strangers with their child and can they trust them to understand and respect their stormy feelings? This distrust will be reflected not only by questions about fees but also by questions as to the age, training, and experience of the worker and of the psychiatrist and psychologist who will be working with the child. Personal questions will be asked, such as whether the worker has children and what problems he encounters in his own family life. However, questions about money and how the worker deals with these questions in terms of his ethical values are especially important because some parents consider this area as the most vulnerable.

> *Case Example:* Mr. T. discussed the fee for the study and wondered if we could bill him for it as a charge that took place several months before, so he could claim it as an income tax deduction. When I stated that we could not alter the date of the actual examination, he then wondered if he could give the fee as a contribution to the clinic and thus deduct it as a donation to a nonprofit organization. When this was refused as a possibility, he explained that his insurance company would pay the fee anyway, and if we wished we could raise the total costs since it would not come out of his pocket and there was no reason not to make a reasonable profit. When I reviewed the fee in terms of his essential ability to pay according to his income, he spoke of the great trust and confidence he had in us; but soon it was obvious that he could trust no one, not his company, his wife, or his child. His face was bitter as he related the humiliation he felt when others looked at him, for they must think, "That man has a crazy child."

As the parents are asked to sign the forms for release of information, attitudes toward confidential matters emerge, such as feelings of distrust and discomfort at the thought of exposure; anxiety is expressed as to which people are to see the child and whether they are professionally competent. All of these are clues to the parents' own feelings. These become the guideposts along which the worker feels his way, allowing the parents to lead him until it is safe for him to take over direction and guidance after certain paths have become clear.

As the study begins, the worker also begins to think of its termination. He holds in his mind an end point around which cluster such questions as these: What goals and expectations do the parents have? Are these realistic and possible in view of the child's illness? What psychic strengths do the parents have? What resources does the clinic have to help them and what other resources exist in the community? How will it be possible to bring these and other such questions one by one into the study proper, so that they do not suddenly loom up at the end as being hastily and abruptly considered? Indeed, these questions are the major realities and reveal sources of feelings and conflicts, which become, then, the issues for discussion and for speeding the study forward.

SEPARATE INTERVIEWS

After the joint hour with the parents, interviews proceed with each of them alternately. This sequence may be interrupted for any special needs, and joint interviews may also take place as need for these arises during the course of the study.

For the sake of convenience, we will discuss some of the possible content of the interviews, keeping in mind that it is impossible to say that such and such occurs in the first hour, the second, or the third. Some parents quickly express the total problem in the very first interview, and others approach it slowly, revealing the problem to its deepest extent and complexity only as they proceed. Still others present the problem in pieces and fragments, leaving out essentials, proceeding elliptically, or expressing themselves in a confused and disorderly way.

In the first hour, the mother or father may be anxious about the one-to-one relationship. Neither the marital partner nor other members of the family are present to divide the worker's glances and attention. Nor are they present to give protection, to blame, or to share the task of exploration. Momentarily there may seem to be nothing to say and the pauses may be uncomfortable. On the other hand, there is a relief about being able to express freely what one thinks without the inhibiting presence of the marital partner. At times, feelings of disloyalty arise, guilt about expressing anger toward the husband or wife, and fears that the worker will misconstrue these feelings or betray them when the other partner is next seen. The swift identification and clarification of these feelings are part of the worker's activity and essential for enhancing a clear flow of feelings and information so necessary for diagnostic clarity.

When a wife speaks of her husband, it may be to reveal intense marital conflict, perhaps to project their child's problem on him, or to express concern that their child's problem is overwhelmingly difficult for her husband and will cause his breakdown. Regardless of what is behind the content or the manner of presentation, she is speaking of herself, and it is to this fact that the worker must be attuned. He cannot, and indeed dare not, join with the wife in understanding her husband's motives. Apart from the likelihood that she would tell her husband of the worker's sympathetic response—probably angering and frightening him away—such an action would simply bulwark her defense against understanding her own feelings about her child and the part played by her feelings in this study, which is the central business above everything else. It is most painful to speak of one's own feelings and far easier to speak of a husband's and child's motives. Content, therefore, is best utilized when the worker takes from it what is obviously the wife's and mother's own feeling. He reflects her feelings back to her and helps her to see that these involve her own troubled concern. In this way she becomes aware that the purpose of the worker's interviews with her is to help her gradually to understand her feelings—what they are and what they mean—and on the basis of this knowledge come to understand how they will shape and influence the decisions which will come at the end of the study.

There is a natural reluctance to undergo this process. It means a great deal of hard work and each hour involves a heavy emotional and physical strain. Resentment and fear of the responsibility are also present. Alone in the interview room, the parent may feel uniquely isolated, bad, helpless. Despite, perhaps, achievements in professional, business, social, or family life, the mother may feel weak and helpless, and her accomplishments in the face of this "failure" with her child may seem insignificant. As a result, she may attack the clinic and the worker, as well as her child and her husband, and demand answers of the "expert" as to what to do. Accompanying the wish for answers is the anxiety that they will be neither pleasant nor desirable. While the mother may express happiness over the scrupulous attention being shown their problem, she may also fear that the hours of time devoted to the study will uncover angry feelings, mean thoughts, and guilts which will confirm her as a poor, inadequate individual who is primarily responsible for the family's difficulties.

She has the same mixed feelings about her husband's participation. On the one hand, she is glad that for the duration of the evaluation his exclusive attention will be on her and the child and that during those evening hours after the child is asleep they will have time to discuss and share their daytime experiences. Many couples comment, in fact, on the value of this concentrated focus on themselves and their child because it directs attention to a problem around which their feelings were hidden or denied. On the other hand, she may feel frightened of her husband's intense participation, his scrutiny not only of his relationship to their child but to her—an examination in which judgment may go against her.

Case Example: Mrs. D. is a thin, plain-featured woman of fifty who dressed in a prim, spinsterish fashion. Her voice quavered as she spoke of being an adopted child and never knowing her real parents. She married Mr. D. five years after he had lost his first wife. She was almost thirty-six then and had given up thoughts of marriage until she met him. He was reluctant to marry her and only did so because he needed someone to care for his two children. She doubted whether he ever loved her. When she became pregnant with Henry, to her own great surprise, dismay, and apprehension, her husband was shocked and angry. She had thoughts of her son's being born defective, damaged, because of doubts and fears concerning the morality of her own real mother and the possibility that her real father might have been trash. Fearful thoughts were also present that her real father might have had syphilis, transmitted through her blood to Henry and causing his present epilepsy. Her husband never accepted Henry, never was close to him, and paid more attention to his first wife's children. She had been afraid, at first, that when they came here her husband would insist on Henry's going to a state institution. She would never stand for that. She was surprised that her husband expressed guilt at the clinic for his previous rejection of Henry and his thoughts of divorcing her. Now he wants to do whatever he can to help and to get the best treatment possible for her son.

First Hour with the Father

For many fathers the first hour with the worker alone heralds a deeper participation than ever before. Some fathers welcome this to a certain extent, recognizing its logic and rightness. They complain of having been shut out of previous efforts at help or of not recognizing until now the deep considerations which must involve them. A psychiatric study may call for change of a radical nature for the family—change involving much expenditure of time and money and sometimes even a move to a new place in order to obtain the help a child needs.

But there are other vital reasons for the father's involvement. He plays a major part in giving consistency and continuity to family life: consistency in the love he gives to his wife, so that she can give steadily to the child, and continuity from his being always present and available as a source of strength and economic security. His presence for the evaluation is a continuation of this support to his wife and child. Without his presence, the mother and child are incomplete, the understanding they achieve is incomplete, and the decisions they make lack the necessary power and authority. These are in addition to the incomplete picture the team would obtain should the father be absent. Each member of the family would be sensitive to his absence. In his interviews with the team, the child, from his various levels of awareness, comments on the importance of his father's presence. The mother, confronted with the presence of her husband each day of the study and sensitive to his reactions as he participates, tells much that is revealing of their relationship. But the father—often showing annoyance and constantly reacting to his wife's and child's presence in this confused situation—begins to discover for himself as he examines his relationships what his part has been in family life, along with how he pictures and thinks about his wife and child and how he imagines they think of him.

> *Case Example:* Mr. G. said it was very difficult to understand Martin, his son. He and his wife were not able, apparently, to do the right things for him. He felt Martin was lazy, that he would not do what he was capable of doing. He found it difficult to think that it might be a family problem. He and his wife have had words on this score. She thinks Martin is disturbed and should be treated gently and that Mr. G. is too harsh with the child. He described the disciplinary problem at home and said he was often put into the position of having to punish the child. His wife asks Martin a dozen times to do something without results, and then as the father he has to take over. His wife is too permissive and indecisive. He described himself as a man of action who expects an order to be followed when he gives it.
>
> He then described at length his professional and business activities, his successes, his hopes for the future, and his hopes for his son to help him. His father had been an old military man, born in Germany, and extremely strict. He does not want to raise his son the same way he had been raised, but he wants him to know order and discipline. He spent some time comparing his own childhood with Martin's. He used to go mountain climbing and had a gang, but Martin plays alone, and he recalls Martin as a young child playing with toys like a little girl. The amount of time and attention his wife gives to Martin is very great and he has noticed this

particularly here at the hotel. His wife picks up after Martin, practically dresses him; this disgusts him and he finds himself trying to control his anger, not only with Martin, but with his wife. This is why, he guessed, they both think of him as harsh. Martin does come between them. This is due to his clinging to his mother, not having friends, complaining that he does not get along, acting as if "What's the use? Just chuck the whole thing." When the worker commented that perhaps Mr. G. felt like this about the study, he agreed. He thought it was important for him to be here despite the "awful Kansas weather," because everything he has tried has been "stymied," and they need help.

In all likelihood the mother's major source of concern is her children, for they are her central responsibility. This is true even if she is employed or running a business or engaged in a profession. Even if she gives over this responsibility to household help, it is culturally expected that she will maintain control of the children's care by closely supervising those to whom she gives this assignment. The father's central responsibility, however, is divided between his family and making a living. Without a doubt, the father feels the illness of his child as a blow to his sense of adequacy, to his success as a father and as a man. He takes pride in his children as reflections of his manliness, his potency, and when they do well in school and in the community, they further reflect him and bolster his social status. In the first hours of the study, the father will quickly reveal what coming to the clinic means to his status and to his feelings about himself. In the case example given above, Mr. G. indicated quickly that he was successful in his profession and that his orders were quickly obeyed. This not uncommon type of defense was his way of pointing out that in one area, at least, he was successful and deserved to be respected.

The worker must be aware of the father's numerous anxieties when he participates and the varied forms of expression these may take. But no matter in what form or style the anxieties are expressed, the worker must clarify those in particular that prevent an accommodation to the study, to participation and involvement, and to coming to grips with the child and his disruptive influence on the family. Thus, the worker may comment gently on the fact that coming to the clinic makes the father unhappy and frightened, doubtful of his success in other fields, and feeling that he might possibly be depreciated here and not respected; but these feelings are called to his attention only to help him participate wholeheartedly in the study rather than to modify his character structure or to examine his personality traits.

The manner in which the worker promotes the father's adjustment to the study is influenced by a complexity of factors. In general, workers are not yet too comfortable about dealing with fathers. Insistence on their presence has been a relatively recent development in clinic practice. Many rationalizations were developed by hospitals and clinics to explain why fathers could not be involved. They were too busy at work and too uninvolved in family life, since their major task was to earn money and keep the family economically secure. The mother was considered the primary factor in the child's disturbance, and, therefore, any essential change for the better had to take place in the mother-child relationship. But such false reasoning, used frequently by the fathers themselves, often concealed the workers' reluctance to complicate a process already difficult to fathom. It also concealed the workers' uneasiness about status and competitiveness that the father caused by an aggressive, challenging approach to the relationship; thus, doubts and questions were raised in their minds about their own capacities and achievements. Fathers, they found, are also frequently action-oriented, contemptuous of feelings and introspection, and insistent upon cold, hard facts. These generalizations about fathers often blinded the worker to the fact, that, like the mother, the father is extremely sensitive about his place in the family and deeply concerned about the part he plays in the problem, even though at first he may conceal this intense involvement.

When the worker is not frightened by the often imposing presence of fathers (and, of course, a good many present themselves not as powerful but as withdrawn and weak), he can see beyond their defenses to the feelings involved and deal directly

with such absurdities as, "I know nothing about the child because
I am never home," or "My wife can tell you much more because
she knows the child better," or "Men know nothing about such
things." If the worker regards the father's evasions as offensive or
views them as a refusal to cooperate or as an attack against his
professional capacities, he misses their true significance, and becomes preoccupied instead with his own hurts. When the parents
sense these feelings in the worker, as well as the inconsistency and
uncertainty of his professional approach, the process falters. Rather,
the worker should acknowledge the father's efforts and success on
his job, his achievement in supplying the family with material
needs, the hard work he has contributed, and the natural limits
of his time with his family. But the worker should also proceed
to show interest in the father's observations, his thoughts, and his
deductions as to the causes of the problem. He should state, clearly,
simply, and directly, that the father has naturally been affected by
the troubles of his child, that no person, in fact, could help but be
worried. He also stresses the point that the father's observations and
point of view will be helpful to the study and of value to the child,
the mother, and, above all, to himself. His approach to the father,
then, is that he is a sensitive, intelligent, and perceptive person who
is being asked, perhaps, to think along unusual paths or in unaccustomed ways but who is capable of doing so after some exer-
cises in that direction and with encouragement and assistance.
Thus, the worker might say, "Since you must have given lots of
thought to why your child behaves in this way, think with me
about it," or "Tell me more about the circumstances in which this
particular incident happened, because you feel it is important and
you may very well be right." Above all, the worker seeks details
because they contain feelings, which are the heart of the matter
and when released flow forth to give facts dimension and illumina-
tion. As a result, the parent is often astonished that one event, one
detail, or one fact may convey many different feelings and many
new ideas about a situation. It becomes an amazing experience for
him, then, to continue an exploration that promises to give insight
into problems which before seemed narrow, enclosed, barren, and
insoluble.

Case Example: Mr. W. was angry that his son required residential treatment. He wanted him to go to a private boarding school. In the future, he said, when his son became an adult, the relationships he formed in private boarding school would endure, and he would have lasting friendships. The friends he would make there would be interesting and fascinating, whereas in public high school he would make no lasting friendships. The worker did not question this view but wondered whether other differences between a private boarding school and residential treatment bothered Mr. W. besides those he had expressed. Mr. W. was thoughtful for a moment and then stated that his son's being in residential treatment meant that he was still ill and a patient rather than a student. The worker commented that this was true, and in residential treatment the parents were in a different relationship to their son. He agreed. "In a residential treatment center, it means that I am not his father. Others take this away from me, or at least I have to share this responsibility. I guess that does bother me. In a private school, I am still the parent, at least, more than if he is in treatment, and then he does what I want him to do. I don't like his being dependent on treatment, using it as a crutch."

The parent, in this instance, has arrived at some understanding of what it means for him to have his son in treatment, and one fact—his son's need for residential treatment—unfolded to reveal a number of feelings that enlarged and enriched this whole area.

The worker need not give involved technical explanations about the purpose of the study. Inevitably, when these are offered, the worker uses technical jargon, and even if he presents them with great clarity, it is usually to clarify his own thoughts about the process rather than to make them useful to the parents. It is also dubious whether the parent is prepared to listen intently, engaged as he is in grappling with his own anxieties. If he should hear what the worker does say, he may emphasize the wrong thing or let his own fears dictate what is important. In this case, the worker may not become immediately aware of what is taking place or may miss what has happened altogether, because, instead of listening, he is talking and explaining. When the worker does speak, it should be at the point where the parent seems most alert, most keenly attuned to what is being said, and where the rapport between the worker and the parents is so close that a comment serves to quickly hook thoughts together, and the relationship as well. Thus, the worker guards against being too subtle and proceeding too rapidly with insights which are his own and from which the parent is as yet at some distance.

Technique is impoverished and insufficient when it utilizes a heavy hand and is authoritatively and conspicuously prominent. It requires a light touch to be unobtrusive; in other words, the worker must be so familiar with the tools of his trade that they are a part of him. He is not too preoccupied then to give the parent the freedom to say what needs to be said, to express all that he can. Out of this freedom to use everything available to them, the worker and the parents can sift through to the heart of the problem.

The worker is always aware that he is a stranger or outsider to this family. More than mothers, fathers seem to resent having to "wash dirty linen in public"; a man should be strong enough to resolve his own problems. He may feel his first loyalty is to his wife and child, and to express anger and disappointment about them is to fail them; he may think that to confide in a stranger shows preference for the outsider and, therefore, is traitorous. In this event, the worker points out quite directly that this reaction is still another quite natural fear of involvement and of revealing oneself. Such feelings may even go back to the ingrained tradition implanted since childhood that one does not "tattle" and a family's affairs are secret and not to be repeated outside. When a child violates this dictum he risks his parents' disapproval; undoubtedly as a grown man, the father will project this same feeling onto the worker, wanting and sensing approval for talking but not sure whether the worker genuinely likes him for it. The worker does well to guard this loyalty and to point out that he does not wish to "divide and conquer" the father's family. He points out further that the father's exposure of the mother or the child is still a defense unless it is accompanied by a thoughtful exploration into the feelings that the events or interactions he is describing aroused in him and into the connection between his feelings and the family tension. Real disloyalty is the fear of change and resistance to the time required to increase inner understanding.

> *Case Example:* In the beginning of the interview, Mr. D. had some difficulty overcoming his reticence, and was cautious and wary in expressing feelings. He was thinking of placement of the child, he said, but had felt depressed about this. It might sound calloused, but this was the best solution. I said I knew his problem with the child had worried him greatly. He replied that it had, so much so that it had interfered with his career, which had been going pretty well. He described his success in business. His child now overshadows all of this. I commented that his success in business had given him much confidence, but his trouble with his child had made him feel bewildered. He agreed that this was true and said that it was so easy to understand other children and do things with them; they liked him, but not his own son. He began to describe a tense marital situation filled with disagreement and quarrels. He had certain ideas regarding play with the child, discipline, and feeding. Uneasily he stated he might be wrong regarding these things, and he looked carefully at me. He felt he should not attack his wife and child here. I commented on his concern regarding my taking sides, perhaps judging his wife right and him wrong. He agreed. After all, she might be attacking and criticizing him in the same way, and again he peered intently at me. When I commented he seemed to feel that he might be disloyal, but also fearful of what his wife might be saying about him, he agreed. It might be, he thought, that the fault is with him. He is not patient and he is easily angered. His wife wants a great deal from him, but it is hard for him to give in return. He feels that his

son turns away from him; he just fails to get love from him. He is frightened his wife is not well, and he described her taking an overdose of phenobarbital several years ago. She is withdrawn from people, has few friends, does not get along in the community. She is oversensitive about the child, overprotective, and she is a disorganized housekeeper, a poor cook. He has endeavored to make suggestions to her, perhaps not too kindly, but she would accept nothing in any way to do with the child. I commented he seemed to feel shut out from his family. He agreed, and, enlarging on this theme, related that for the past year and a half his wife has slept with the child in the boy's bedroom. He believes this is neither normal nor healthy. Perhaps he has fallen out of love with his wife and she senses this. His marriage has been difficult from the very beginning. It became more evident when their child was born and it seems that he has felt more distant from his wife since then. He wondered why this was so; it had never occurred to him to date their difficulties from that time on. Perhaps his wife had not wanted a child. He should not say that really, but somehow he felt she did not want to be a mother. When I asked why he thought that, he described his wife's moodiness and depression during pregnancy, fear of giving birth, and anger about stopping work. He expressed guilt for revealing this. I commented he felt he was betraying his wife rather than increasing his understanding of the situation and perhaps this was so because I was a stranger to him, and he was not sure what I might think of him. He agreed and then said that the idea of having a child after several years of waiting came as a surprise to him also and, at first, he resented the changes they had to make but he thought he really wanted a family. At the end of the hour, he expressed surprise it had gone so rapidly.

Second Hour with the Mother

Now each participant in the study has experienced some

involvement. The child has indicated and may even have reported to his parents his reactions to the experience, the psychiatrist, and the psychologist. He may have done this directly, telling his parents about them, which one he prefers or whether he likes or dislikes them both. He may have expressed his wish, perhaps with eagerness, to continue or his wish to stop and return home. Of course, he may not have said anything or even refused to say anything about his first contacts. What the mother chooses to reveal in this second hour about the child's reactions, as well as how she obtained or received them, is significant and useful. Every element of her report may be true, but the worker will encourage the mother to go into detail about how she observed her child's reactions in order to determine to what extent this is the case. But the worker adds an interpretation, commenting that these observed reactions in her child might belong to her as well. This comment does not detract from her story, as told, nor does it question its veracity; but it does give the story an added significance. The mother will often use the child by attributing her thoughts to him and will have him serve this function not only because of her close relationship to him but because he is inextricably bound up with her own thoughts and emotions. Further, her use of the child in this way also serves to maintain some distance from the worker, some distance away from his sensing how much she may like or dislike her participation in the study. In making this comment, the worker accepts her report unless it is incoherent and vague, but he also suggests further meanings to help the mother see that she can express her feelings more directly without fear of being criticized.

Some parents are ready to see that their child serves as an avenue to their minds, and that their minds serve as an avenue back to the child. Others may need more time before this kind of recognition is possible; their own personality organization is too tenuous to examine any of their feelings so directly. A discussion, for example, of the child's attitude toward coming for appointments gives them the opportunity to express their own feelings without highlighting them or bringing them boldly out for open scrutiny by the worker.

How does the worker tell how fast to go? Since a majority

of parents can deal rapidly with feelings, the worker can often determine speed by gently touching on feelings about coming to Topeka: "You must have been apprehensive when the doctor told you to come to a psychiatric clinic," or "Your being referred here must have come as a surprise," or "I wonder what your reactions were when the school suggested your child might need psychiatric help." The parents' responses to these tentative leads by the worker reflect their capacity for a direct recognition of their feelings and for dealing with them.

The ways in which the mother receives her impressions and information from the child are illuminating. If she indicates to the worker that she insists on questioning her child as to what he said to the psychiatrist and what the psychiatrist said, the worker can begin to deal with such fears as that the child will expose his parents, that the parents are being kept in the dark, or that the child is undergoing an experience apart from his parents. If the mother does not listen to the child or appears indifferent to his experiences and reactions, the worker notes that this particular mother may be so preoccupied with herself that she fails to notice her child or that she is perhaps inhibited and immobilized out of immense anxiety. If, instead, the mother listens to the child with alertness and sensitivity, making no undue intrusion into what he is undergoing, this may be an important indication of strength and maturity. The worker circles these impressions, seeking ways to help the mother unfold this or that fact, this or that feeling, in order to increase their understanding of the varied meanings of the family situation.

The child may tell his mother that he likes the psychiatrist. The worker, hearing this report, may comment that the mother seems pleased, that it must also be easier for her to come for interviews when she knows her child is happy to see the doctor. The mother may agree that this is so, thus conveying that she feels liked and accepted; however, the mother may possibly wonder why a stranger finds her child lovable when her own feelings toward him are a mixture of anger, fear, love, and hate. Is she thereby a lesser person, a poorer parent than she should be? Her child's liking the psychiatrist and psychologist may build fears in her of his going away from her, with the result that she will lose control over him and his thoughts. Perhaps, she thinks, these people will influence him to leave his parents, to learn values that they will abhor, to receive information about aggression and sex which will be frightening and difficult to suppress. Then, won't her child become more troublesome and more ill than he already is? Thus, the study is often perceived as opening Pandora's box and letting loose uncontrollable behavior, which earlier family life was able to contain.

Case Example: Mrs. G. appeared composed, neatly dressed, almost euphoric in her manner, with an inappropriate cheerfulness. She voluntarily stated she was feeling better because Richard wanted very much to see Dr. F. again. She was pleased that he liked Dr. F. It made her happy that he liked someone other than herself. It made her feel he was capable of liking others, and it might eventually mean for her an easier separation from him. This was said with a cheery belligerence and underlying anger with Dr. F. and Richard. She thought that Dr. F. was overly fond of children. I inquired about her meaning. She thought that it was not easy to like Richard, his behavior was destructive, difficult. He kicked and screamed at the slightest provocation, at the slightest frustration. I commented that it surprised her that Richard could like someone and that someone could find qualities in him to like. She agreed. I suggested that she was both pleased and puzzled by this. She was thoughtful and then said that it seemed he was too much for her, made her angry easily.

She was finding the same thing true of her husband. He has told her he would like to run and turn his back on the whole problem. She was disgusted with him and with his wish to desert at this critical time, although she feels like running also. She is under constant criticism from her in-laws, who accused her of not feeding the child properly, of giving him too much phenobarbital, even though she was following her pediatrician's instructions.

She had also been accused of not disciplining him properly. She felt she had been the victim of confused advice and did not think men and doctors knew their business. When I said she feared that she would not be able to depend on us and I had the impression she was ready to fight us with raised fists just as she had her husband and her in-laws, she laughed and agreed this was so.

But the worker does not focus only on the current aspects of the study and the mother's reactions to these. This would ignore the past and present content of family life and experience, which is so necessary for understanding the child's illness. Indeed, when a parent insists on talking exclusively about the study, she is using it as a device to prevent new understanding. It is as if the parent (usually without awareness) is actually saying, "How can I speak throughout this hour and not once come to grips with painful issues?"

Nevertheless, the way the mother speaks of current events and of her expectations for the study tells a great deal about the past and present home situation and the hopes and expectations of the family for the child. If he is intellectually retarded, his parents often demand that he be of normal intelligence and they wish the study to prove he is. If he is organically damaged, they wish for him to be physically healthy, and that the study should make him so. If he is delinquent and aggressive, they wish the study to make him conforming and compliant, even though their own approach is a conflicting mixture of seductivity, aggression, and compliance.

It is wise to caution at this point that no one pattern in family groups is so clearly etched and delineated that the clinic can dispense with the labor of careful exploration and effort to understand a particular family with all of its unique characteristics. While one pattern may look much like another, it is still different in its texture and color, and the story as it emerges will take a shape never seen before in precisely the same way.

Each parent is encouraged to speak of the present and to connect it with the past. If the content is exclusively from the past, encouragement is given to speak and to recognize current meanings before returning to the past. It is an oscillating process that makes connections between focal points and abscessed areas. These are touched and punctured gently, sometimes by the parent, sometimes with caution by the worker, to release feelings long repressed and smouldering—feelings which if not given freedom will prevent a successful conclusion of the study. The release of these feelings is for the purpose of helping the parent see herself, mainly in terms of the irrational hopes she has for her child, how these influence the expectations of the study, and how these have been and will be unprofitable should they persist. We want to help her understand how painful it is to consider new alternatives to a problem and, although these are consciously desired, how she fears and fights the thought of them. And, finally, we want to help her understand that she need not deal with this conflict by using such young ways of behaving as anger and aggression, immaturity and irrational thought, but, rather, that her desire and strength to help her child, as a mother, is her greatest asset.

Second Hour with the Father

Many of the principles and concepts discussed in relationship to the mother apply equally to the father and need not be repeated. But there are many new, unaccustomed things about the study to which the father may react with some discomfort because of his particular place in the family and his degree of involvement. The mother, most likely, has been the parent who has consulted doctors and guided the child through previous medical procedures. The father is now involved in this process, for this week at least, and he lives in very close proximity to his family. Above all, there are the interview appointments and an unaccustomed way of life at the clinic with an unaccustomed focus on feelings, thoughts, and self. The father becomes aware of many things about his wife and child, their interaction with each other as well as his interaction with them. He may report how difficult his wife finds it to control the child, thus casting light on his own attitudes about permissiveness and controls and on the course of action he has assumed or failed to assume earlier in the area of relationships. He may become more aware of how frightening it is for his wife to be a mother, thus

revealing what his thoughts are about being a father. The picture
he presents of the child's behavior will give glimpses of his thoughts
about the development of the child, about aggression, competition,
sexuality, and his concerns and expectations for the child's growing
up.

In the course of the interview, he may experience a further
deepening of feelings about involvement in this or any possible
future process.

> *Case Example:* The father, a pharmacist, stated in a
> tight-lipped way that he would do for his son whatever
> was necessary. When the worker commented that it
> sounded as if he were saying that he would take his
> medicine, the father grinned and agreed, showing some
> warmth and relaxation from his grimness. He saw his age
> as preventing change and found it difficult to come here
> and at the same time think of his work. In his work, he
> said, he sees many sick people, people who have heart
> conditions, multiple sclerosis, muscular dystrophy, and he
> could not grieve over everyone with these illnesses. If he
> tried, he would be unable to work. He did not think he
> could pull himself together again, not after he went
> through taking himself apart.

This particular father shows much anxiety about participation, but this is a frequent phenomenon. He is frightened of what
he may learn about his wife, his child, and himself, as well as how
the worker will value him. If the worker is aware of these fears and
deals with each revelation as it emerges, not as evidence, not as
simply the accumulation of mountains of facts, or as a penetration
of defenses but, instead, as an enlargement of knowledge and respect
between himself and the father, then the father will find the process
valuable and be less afraid of exposing himself to himself and the
worker. Thus, in the example above, if the worker sensitively comments on the father's distaste for his part in the study in language
quite familiar to his ears, the parent will usually be able to give

illuminating details about the feelings he needs to master in order to involve himself.

After the worker has seen the parents together and separately for several hours, he begins to sift through the material in order to make the first organized and systematic presentation of it to the other team members. This is not his first communication to others, since he has spoken to them before about the case, often in the corridors, at coffee, and in brief moments between appointments. Although this quick, informal sharing of impressions has advantages, it may also lead to poor results. For example, the worker, the psychologist, or the psychiatrist may give tentative impressions which the other team members take as definite and perhaps act on prematurely in their individual processes, to the detriment of the study. Thus, a psychologist might tell his team that a child appears to be severely retarded, and then later, when assessing his material, arrive at a different conclusion. Or the worker may think he heard the psychologist make this statement but had not found the time to check. In turn, the worker may present a somber, pessimistic picture of the parents and their strength to the psychiatrist, causing him to judge the child against an environmental background which offers little support or warmth. What does seem to get communicated at these times, then, is the natural anxiety of the team members, each eager to give some picture of the difficult problems confronting him.

But for this first team conference, the worker must organize his material to meet a number of important requirements. First, he must arrange his material for his own benefit, to see in an orderly fashion what total picture is developing in the process, and what patterns of knowledge and understanding are forming to increase his understanding of a particular family. Secondly, he must select the important facts and observations the psychologist needs to be aware of in order to continue psychological tests with a better understanding of a child's past and current experiences. The psychologist should know, for example, that five years before this study the child had psychological tests which placed him in the average range of intelligence and then later received successively lower scores on several other tests. He should know whether the child is taking current tests without the medication to which he has been accustomed for a long period of time. If the parents note that their child functions best when limits and controls are firmly placed, this information may also be vital to the test procedures. Third, the worker must give the psychiatrist such significant information as a child's unexplained high temperature in early infancy, followed by a period of restlessness and hyperactivity, or a mother's severe depressive episodes after the birth of her child, making her emotionally unavailable to him for long periods of time. The time available to give such information is limited. The worker cannot take up more than his share of time since this will annoy his team colleagues, who are waiting their turns. This limitation need not be a disadvantage, but it does require a succinct, lucid ordering of material and the worker's giving careful thought to the following items:

1. Why do the parents say they are coming to the clinic and what are the reasons they cite for coming at this particular time, as well as their expressed expectations?

2. What unconscious reasons do the parents have for coming now?

3. What is the present problem as the parents view it?

4. How do I view the deeper problem that I believe the parents do not recognize?

5. What sequence of developmental events has brought the problem to its present critical point?

6. What previous treatment efforts have been made and what are the reasons given by the parents for their failure?

7. Why have previous treatment efforts failed?

8. How would I assess the character and personality of each parent and how these have had and are having their influence upon the child?

9. How are the parents progressing and how are they likely to use the findings of the study and our material and psychological resources, as well as those of the community, to deal with the problem?

As the worker listens to the material that the psychologist and the psychiatrist report, in turn, he notes where it makes inroads on his own material and impressions; it may either enlarge the scope of his understanding about this family, making more clear and sure the path to follow and the areas that must yet be explored, or it may be incompatible with his findings. If the latter, it is imperative that the team should know where the incompatibilities are, what contradictions are present, and why they exist. The preconference may be compared to a large jigsaw puzzle in which the function of the conference members is to put together a great number of facts, insights, impressions, and speculations and to study the results carefully as they go along in order to see what further efforts they must make to achieve a total picture. As the other team members present their findings, the worker is given an opportunity to stand apart from the problem and view his own process in relation to others. What has been amorphous and vague may have become clearer. He now may know how and in what direction to bend his efforts, so he can obtain what he suspected was missing. For example, the fact may emerge that a mother and father were never able to talk about what their child means to them, what they want from him, and how they encouraged him to identify with them, because subtly they had veered away from these aspects of their relationship with him. When the worker places the various parts of his material in logical juxtaposition, an awareness of its deficits will become more likely.

SOCIAL WORKER'S FINAL INTERVIEW

After the first conference, the worker approaches the parents with a larger view of the problem, and with new leads to follow. The type of family situation and problem determines the kind of techniques he should use. For example, certain specific techniques are necessary for dealing with the parents of a retarded or brain-damaged child. Although they are painfully aware of the nature and degree of the illness and of its inevitable effects on the family, their own psychological make-up neither produced the symptom nor continues it. The parents usually wish to deny the existence of the retardation, to reject it, or to overcompensate by exaggerating it as a hopeless condition. They are, nevertheless, dealing with an external event which has happened to them, rather than with profound psychological problems in which their conflicts are enmeshed with those of the child. This latter situation we encounter in a school phobia characterized by the child's inability to separate from his parents. In such an instance, the parents actually may be aggravating the very illness for which they are seeking aid.

Although the parents of a retarded child may surround him with their own deep hurts and unconscious expectations, throw the net of their own guilts and angers over his shoulders, and view him possessively, the fact of the external damage—the retardation—is always apparent. Those feelings that are unrealistic about this can be sorted out from those that are realistic and, therefore, helpful to the child and his family.

> *Case Example:* Mrs. C. was calm and more relaxed today, and the worker shared with her the tentative impression that while her son was severely retarded, as she had expected, he seemed to have potentialities for growth in certain areas. Mrs. C. listened carefully, commenting on how gentle the worker was with her in contrast to the bluntness and crudeness of the first physician who had told her, "Put your child away and forget him." She went on to say, "Those early doctors never went as deep; they never talked about my feelings or cared about me."
>
> Whenever she went anywhere with the child, she was sensitive to the stares of others. She thought they were thinking that she must be defective and damaged. She felt herself getting red and flushed inside and wanted to scream at them. This is why it soon became impossible to take the child outside. She restricted her social life, and even neglected her husband. If he said anything about the child, she would fight him. She said that she knew her child needed another environment but she couldn't help him because she regretted his birth, and she wondered why God had punished the child instead of her alone. It is true she would be lonely without the

boy, but she could solve that problem by working and meeting people again. The last few years had been a waste for her, the child, and, she guessed, her husband also.

While it is not always possible to present the parents with tentative impressions or findings after the preconference, the worker begins to introduce into his last hours of discussion those factors in their situation which will play an important part in shaping recommendations. These concern parental feelings about wishes for help: how do they feel about psychiatric treatment, placement for the child, referral back to their own community, the investment of considerably more time and money, and, finally, further involvement of themselves? An exploration of these questions will alert the parents to the fact that a summing up is under way—a summing up which will point the way to action.

FINAL JOINT CONFERENCE

Before the social worker and the psychiatrist meet with the parents, the former have made a final review together as to whether there is a consensus in regard to the findings and recommendations. Frequently, the staff conference has discussed many difficult and complex issues, some of which remain unresolved, and now the social worker and the psychiatrist need a brief period to integrate the opinions of others with their own thinking. Those controversial and provocative questions that often arise in professional discussions cannot be brought into the meeting with the parents, but should remain for the professional staff to discuss as future issues. The parents will need the worker and the psychiatrist to be clear, convincing, and consistent if they are to strengthen their ability to meet the requirements of the patient for future help. Occasionally, parents who are struggling with great desperation for help, as well as with disillusionment and shock over the patient's illness, seek to control these feelings by attacking any uncertainty or lack of conviction they sense in the team or on the part of the social worker and the psychiatrist as to the findings. As a result, they would discredit the study because it might require too much of them or be greatly disappointing as compared with their initial expectations. There are also times when the child and his family present a diagnostic dilemma which cannot be resolved during the relatively short period of the examination. In such an instance the team must share this dilemma honestly with the family and present it without being defensive.

The appearance of the psychiatrist, a relatively unfamiliar figure to the parents, may revive the anxieties they have shown in the initial hours of the study. The psychiatrist is usually viewed as an imposing and authoritative figure. He has worked closely with the child and he knows not only his secrets but the family's as well. Thus, he is seen as a figure who may empathize exclusively with the child and attack the parents for having done a poor job. In addition, he may be the bearer of disappointing findings, of unexpected and painful news. The parents' reactions may sometimes even startle and disappoint the worker and the psychiatrist who have assumed too quickly that much has been worked through and need not be repeated.

The persistence of conflict is forgotten by the team. Their assumption of understanding and acceptance by the parents reflects wishful thinking quite as irrational as that with which parents themselves sometimes come. If the initial anxieties of the parents again emerge in the final conference, it is because this regressive phenomenon is universal in the face of the powerful impact that the final conference carries. Once aware of this phenomenon, the psychiatrist and the social worker will not be disconcerted by it; instead, they will carefully gear their explanations to the parents' gradual recovery from shock as they sense the team's warmth, support, and empathy.

The psychiatrist will take the lead, presenting the findings not as a finished package but slowly, in pieces. As he proceeds, he will stop to inquire whether the parents understand each point and will pause to deal with any signs of doubt or incredulity. The worker, of course, actively assists him whenever necessary, since from his objective vantage point he is able to observe such parental reactions as anxiety and physical discomfort, having become sensitized to the mother and father in his close work with them.

The psychiatrist uses language of a nontechnical nature, seeking clear and succinct words which crystallize the problem and its treatment. The parents are involved in each step, and the findings he presents are synchronized to their reactions to the patient, the nature of their defense patterns and their particular anxieties and angers. The parents are encouraged to ask questions and to express their feelings freely. Explanations are given to help them recognize and accept the patient's real illness. These explanations are also based on their relationship with the team, which has been developed to help them express highly charged feelings. If a parent is too compliant and conveys few or no ambivalent feelings, he may be using this acquiescence as a means of escaping from the pain he actually feels from the findings of the study. The team shares the findings in such a way as to release the parents' strengths still further, to get them to consider the resources they genuinely have for dealing with the problem as it is defined, to sum up what they have been able to do for their child rather than what they have not done, and to weigh what insights and knowledge they can bring to bear on deciding a future course.

The presentation of recommendations is a complex task depending on the individual needs of the case. In some instances, the parents are given a recommendation which offers no alternatives. The findings may clearly point to one solution only if the team believes that any other would show a neglect of professional responsibility. Such an instance might be one in which the child desperately needs hospitalization and if he is not immediately hospitalized may be a menace to himself and to others.

A second possible kind of recommendation is to present alternatives, with the team assisting the parents to weigh carefully the advantages and disadvantages of each, as well as the resources they have to use for each course of action. Together, they then arrive at a decision as to what procedure best meets the need of the child and the family.

A third possibility is to present no recommendations because there are no clear-cut avenues to pursue. The team, however, helps to select a course of action which they feel, from their understanding of the findings, most able to pursue.

But no matter what course of action the team decides to follow, the parents continue to be involved in a slow and painstaking struggle to deal with the findings. This struggle may continue with the worker alone after the psychiatrist leaves the conference. If the parents have established a strong relationship with the worker, they may then feel more free to express their doubts about the findings and make use of this final opportunity to show their resistance to them. Other parents will use the opportunity to further the relationship with the worker and even bring out additional insights about their relationship with the patient.

In the meantime, the psychiatrist may see the child for a final good-bye and discuss with him the implications of the findings, having already told the parents that he will do so. Many parents are touched by the consideration and humaneness of the study, the careful attention given to their feelings, and, now in this good-bye, to the feelings of the child. But it may not be the final conference for the parents, since many choose to stay for an extra day or two for further discussions on the findings until they have a clearer understanding of them. The study is not finished until this understanding is achieved, whether at the official close of their visit or months or years later as their thinking matures with time.

CHAPTER III

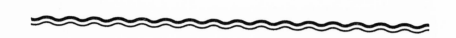

Evaluation of Treatability

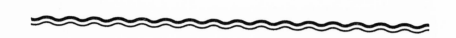

S electing a sound treatment plan for
a child and his parents is often extremely difficult. Since the symptoms alone do not necessarily reflect the severity of the child's underlying disturbance or the degree to which his development is blocked, the treatment methods and goals must be planned individually for each child and his family according to the specific dynamic-genetic diagnosis, whether the symptoms are minimal or

marked (Group for the Advancement of Psychiatry, 1957). To integrate the thinking of all the co-workers involved in an evaluation and to communicate this thinking in an effective way so that the plan of help is useful for both the parents and the child assume that certain principles for the treatment of children have continually been the basis for the diagnostic study. The team diagnostic process leads to an evaluation of the strengths as well as the pathology in the child, the family, and the environment. How the child struggles with his developmental tasks, how he adapts to threats in his growth experiences, and what mechanisms—healthy and unhealthy—he uses in the areas of adjustment are the focus of the evaluation itself.

In particular, we need to evaluate the relation of present difficulties or symptoms and their intensity to the current developmental stage.

> *Case Example:* Melinda was an immature, prepubertal, mildly brain-damaged, and unattractive girl who had no friends, was retarded in school, very self-depreciating, and hostile at home; she was considered by one examiner to be getting considerable gratification from displaying her inadequacy. Along with the reactions to frustration caused by her neurological difficulties and her family's failure to understand these, she was experiencing the conflicts, doubts, and anxieties typical for prepuberty children. The fact that a considerable part of her disturbance was appropriate for her developmental phase suggested that she would be responsive to help with these normal problems as a preparation for help with more severe problems.

In making a diagnosis, we are not merely classifying the child's complex set of symptoms or behavior disorder; we are always exploring ways of helping him. Is it likely that the child can be restored to normal or near normal functioning at home, at school, and in the community? Will the child be able to move freely in the community with only the self-protective selectivity actually required by his vulnerabilities? Or is the child likely to be able to participate only with sustained support? Or is the child so damaged, handicapped, or ill that he can be managed only in a protected environment? Are the implicit aims to facilitate total recovery or to prepare the child and his family for long-time residential care?

During an evaluation, one needs to decide about the child's and the parents' readiness to sustain a therapeutic process on a realistic level.

> *Case Example:* George was an adopted son with a slightly below-average IQ, eight years old, who suffered acutely from the competition of two bright, attractive younger sisters born after he was adopted. Confused, feeling rejected, he was fighting for attention and love in many destructive ways. His attention span was poor and his schoolwork inadequate even in relation to his intelligence quotient of 85. His parents had concluded that he was retarded and should be institutionalized. They did, in fact, reject him so completely that the idea of a major expense for residential therapy with a view to rehabilitating him and his relations to each of his parents was unacceptable. What they had wanted from the evaluation was a recommendation for institutionalization, and they were unwilling to consider any alternative or to make a serious effort to see what progress he might be able to make with therapy.

Allen (1942) lists four interacting evaluations to judge. These include (1) the evaluation of the gestalt of the family constellation; (2) the evaluation of the depth of the family involvement in the child's problems; (3) the evaluation of the child's internalization of the problem as he adapts both to his own needs and those of his family; and (4) the evaluation of the child and his problem in relation to community attitudes and resources. Thus, one tries to evaluate not only what help is needed but also what configuration of factors will allow the family and the child to use that help.

> *Case Example:* Nancy was the much-loved seven-year-

old daughter of an overstimulating, seductive father and
an unstable mother, who tried to keep her beautiful child
a baby or a pet. Her religiously fanatical grandmother
made excessively rigid demands for model behavior. Alternating between angry, aggressive outbursts considered
"wicked" at home, and sad, compliant, but extremely
withdrawn behavior at school, and obsessed by bizarre
fantasies, she was on the verge of a psychotic break.

Nancy herself responded to her contacts with psychiatrist and psychologist during evaluation and wanted
help. Would her parents, dominated by the disapproving
grandmother and deeply entrenched in disturbing ways
of handling Nancy, be able to cooperate? This question
must be evaluated before a plan can be made. (Basically
devoted to Nancy, they finally did decide to put her needs
ahead of those of the grandmother.)

To Allen's list of considerations we can add the question
as to whether the child has ever functioned at a moderately well-
integrated level.

Case Example: John was a violent boy of ten, disturbed
and disturbing in behavior, thought, and feelings. During
evaluation he climbed up porches, onto roofs, throwing
down roof tiles and breaking windows. He seemed more
like an angry, wounded animal than a human child.
Other extremely disturbed children had been greatly
helped by residential care and therapy. What possibilities
were there for him? Scrutiny of his developmental history
showed that he had never had a period of any degree of
equilibrium; he had been an unstable, unresponsive,
angry, screaming, colicky baby with no foundation for well-
being or capacity to settle into a comfortable routine. His
family was desperate for help and able to afford the most
complete treatment possible. He was cautiously accepted
as an inpatient on a trial basis and was given all possible
help. But his total lack of impulse control, of capacity to

relate to a helping person, or to develop greater integration interfered with progress.

Pollak (1952) emphasizes five considerations that are always inherent in treatability: The first consideration is the degree of modifiability of all persons exercising pathogenic influences upon the growth determinants of the child. Second, it is necessary to predict the type of social interaction which the personality development of the patient during therapy probably will produce among other family members. Special attention must be paid to the possibility of creating conflict between parent and child which might result in negative interaction between them. (This is especially likely in patients coming from a narrowly restrictive religious subculture.) Third, each particular disturbance must be recognized as being the result of a constellation of factors and thus can usually be at least partially relieved by working with some of them. Fourth, the forces conducive to health must be considered since often they can also be trusted to operate outside the therapeutic relationship; as a result the child may need help only to overcome his disturbance to the point at which he can use these resources. Fifth, treatment must be recognized as a process which can perhaps be accomplished with different degrees of success, so that even partial removal of incapacitation, or partial emotional relief may be considered a therapeutic gain. The range of possible treatment that the staff envisions will affect the judgment of treatability; closely related to these are the range and flexibility of goals the team is willing to consider.

Case Example: Billy was a disturbed, angry, hyperactive, five-year-old boy whose kindergarten teacher could not cope with him. She persuaded the mother to try to get help for him. The evaluation found his parents in the midst of angry struggles over a divorce, each one fighting for the child's allegiance. One point of view emphasized the impossibility of real therapeutic progress with a child so beleaguered by family conflict. Another point of view emphasized that since the boy had been responsive to examiners during evaluation and was obviously capable of a therapeutic relationship, a salvaging or holding operation would be worth while. The main aim would be to provide support and a relationship favorable to growth during the period of his parents' battles. After the divorce was final and custody was established, further therapy could be undertaken if necessary. This point of view prevailed. And the boy made active use of supportive therapy for considerable individuation, clarification of his sex role, and progress in relating to peers. This relieved the intensity of his dependence on his parents and reduced the impact of their struggles.

The emphasis by Pollak is applicable to the problems in our clinic, if it is remembered that in our sample of cases with approximately 50 per cent of organic problems, pathology is more complex than is implied in the term *psychopathology*. Thus, thinking about possibilities for treatment includes thinking about the integration of medical treatment, environmental controls and activities, and education along with psychotherapy or psychoanalysis.

In the case of the brain-damaged child we cannot hope to "make the child completely normal." What we can do is (1) reduce the overlay of conflict, anger, discouragement, or even despair which have accumulated in reaction to the many real frustrations, (2) help the child see himself as a human being with problems to be solved rather than as a queer rejected person, and (3) help the child understand his limitations more clearly and develop better ways of coping with them, as well as using his resources for the greatest compensation. In such cases we think of combined educational and psychotherapeutic treatment with the goal of freeing the child's positive potentialities while bearing the burden of his limitations.

Those doing an evaluation of the problems which the troubled child presents need the opportunity as well as the objectivity to evaluate the diagnostic process itself. It is easy to see how the evaluation might encounter serious difficulties because of the excessive zeal of the examiners who may consciously or unconsciously visualize the goal of the therapeutic effort as being the complete resolution of personality conflict. Often this ideal goal may be impossible to achieve in practice and may reflect a lack of recognition of the fact that conflicts contain not only pathogenic elements, but also elements conducive to health. The same stubbornness that creates trouble in a disturbed child may benefit him when he resolves enough conflict to use this stubbornness as strength.

The fundamental principle involved here is that human need must be met in the way it presents itself and on its own level of experience. "Depending on the nature and degree of the child's psychopathology and strengths, varying intensities of therapeutic work in particular areas of conflict might be indicated. The specific psychotherapeutic methods may be planned to emphasize one or more aspects of the treatment process: the abreaction of feeling while the child is revealing directly or symbolically his conflicts and defenses; the working through of inner conflicts within the relationship by the development of some insight through the clarification of dynamic patterns and the interpretation of genetic factors; and the strengthening of ego functions through re-education and through the ultimate resolution of illogical attitudes in the therapeutic relationship (Group for the Advancement of Psychiatry, 1957)."

It always has to be realized that organic deficits of any kind increase the child's need to depend on his parents; not only does he experience the usual developmental frustrations and problems but also those created by his handicap, as well as anxiety and resentment over his parents' concern about these failures. All of these things, along with adding to normal dependency, tend to heighten normal developmental anxiety, including separation anxiety; this is precisely because of the child's genuine need for parental help and support, as well as because of more deeply internalized symbiotic patterns rooted in the mutual anxiety of the parents and the child. The same process contributes to intensified aggression in the preoedipal years, and the separation anxiety, the aggression, and the realistic dependence interfere with normal progress of oedipal relationships and normal individuation and eventually progress into latency. Thus, the damaged child is often still embedded in an infantile relationship.

The team process of diagnosis has focused on a study of the child's interactions with his environment since these findings must be seen in relation to his total developmental data. That is, the interaction of constitutional factors in the growth pattern with maturing biological drives must be studied in relation to the pattern of the child's dependence on his parents. Team members try to synthesize the child's physical, emotional, familial, and social difficulties, and to see their relationship to each other. They also assess the child's ways of handling these difficulties and the constitutional resources he can use. It is as important to discover the child's strengths as it is to recognize his weaknesses and the areas of damage that set limitations. Since the team can obtain a true picture of the child only by first helping him to participate to the limit of his capacity, the study clearly must provide not only insights into the child but as much therapeutic benefit as possible for him. This therapeutic result emerges from the child's experience of new satisfactions and from new glimpses of achievements and possibilities for recognition and rewarding relationships. His capacity for such response contributes to the estimate of treatability.

As was stressed in the chapter on the work with parents in the diagnostic examination of children, a major part of the diagnostic work is concerned with helping the parents with those feelings that have deterred them from seeking constructive solutions to the problems of their child. As stated, the team's task is to help parents see what their child means to them, what his difficulties mean to them, what hidden satisfactions and frustrations they have experienced in their struggle with the child, and what the illness means to the child himself. Every effort is made to help the parents look at themselves realistically and honestly. Warm understanding is offered to sustain them in the difficult task of giving up the defenses they have developed to handle their troubled feelings about the way in which the child has disturbed their lives and their guilty feelings over their own contributions to his difficulties. Since the most expert diagnosis can be rendered valueless by the parents' inability to accept it, evaluations of the child, the parent-child relationship, the parent-parent relationship, and the social and cultural setting must provide not only an organized account of the child's development and his problem but also the experience which will allow both parents and child to risk seeking help. It is through the therapeutic handling of the parents' and the child's anxiety in the evaluative process and through their increased understanding of historical factors that the parents and the child become aware of their roles in the family, and gain sufficient confidence in the help recommended to decide eventually to seek a remedy.

In evaluating treatability the team needs to consider that the child's problems have arisen not only in an interpersonal milieu, but in reference to a series of interactions which have evoked a feeling of helplessness or vulnerability, and the emotional or behavioral disability has resulted from the child's struggle to deal with his anxiety. The child not only repeatedly tries to reduce his anxiety over the external threats he feels but secretly contemplates retaliating against them and the person he thinks is responsible for them. Both the child and the family are caught in a repetitive, circular struggle. Every child inevitably has to learn to cope with some frustration; this effort can promote growth and mastery if the task is within his capability. However, it is only when the parent-child relationships have been reasonably good that the child can utilize as challenges to growth the frustrations and threats that he experiences and thus develop inner strength. In the diagnostic process the team evaluates the child's attempts to meet the threats to development and the failures in these. In evaluating ego strength and weakness, and the multiple factors in both, we see not only the unevenness and imbalance in the different aspects of ego development. We also see that continued maturation and continued mastery of developmental tasks can be fostered by the child's achieving from each new phase of personality development some appropriate and realistic satisfactions that help him proceed to the next stage in this development. If we then weigh the range of those satisfactions and achievements against those he has missed, we can plan more clearly for the next steps.

There are important differences to be considered in evaluating the treatability of children as compared with that of adults, even though we can agree that no *absolute* difference exists between such evaluations. Still, a specific recognition must always be made of the child's immaturity and constantly changing developmental level, since these not only influence the nature and intensity of his problems and his reactions to them but also influence the type of relationship he develops with the examiners and the kinds of defenses he uses. Not only are a child's symptoms determined by many mixed factors but they arise from and reflect his current stage of development as well. The impact of any traumatic experience depends on the developmental phase in which such an experience occurs. Although oversimplification is necessary to make the point clearly, it is obvious that the death of a child's mother has different meanings for him as an infant during the first few days of life, before he recognizes her, than it has at seven months, when he is highly sensitive to strangers and to separation from his mother. Similarly, at five years of age, he may be at the peak of small-boy love, while at eight years he may be secure in his peer group and emotionally far less dependent on her.

In considering the question of age and trauma, Allen (1942) makes the point that the child is being delayed or blocked or disturbed in the midst of the process of self-realization, whereas the adult has achieved this to some degree. Moreover, in children both the resistance to change and the drive to change are greater. In looking at the learning process from this standpoint, Allen remarks that the child always asks in each situation, "Shall I individualize further or shall I give the same response as before?" Although the adult has certain established patterns, the child is always faced with the need to initiate and sustain change. Moreover, if disturbance is severe, the child is threatened with the possibility that he will never "grow up." This happens in those instances of psychogenic retardation when a child who with therapy might be able to take his place in the world is institutionalized.

The diagnostic evaluation which attempts to evaluate treatability must recognize that not only do the child's conflicts and his psychopathology require solution but his normal developmental needs must also be met. This requires the possibility of restitution for experiences missed. If the infantile experience has not laid an adequate foundation for basic, healthful narcissism and trust, the development of these is the first prerequisite for further growth. Similarly, if normal foundations have not been laid for the autonomy necessary for early individuation, restitution at this level is essential. The child cannot evolve the appropriate responses for a given developmental level without this kind of rebuilding. Treatability, then, includes the question whether the child will be capable of the healthful and useful regression required for this rebuilding without the total disintegration of his personality.

The use of play in an evaluative study can often provide a glimpse of the child's wishes or hopes, as well as his angry reactions to pressures from adults, competition from siblings, or fears of his own wild impulses. This further exploration of the child's problem and his implied feelings about his own adjustment can provide the opportunity for him to talk about his future and his reaction to the possibility of getting help. His response contributes to the team's judgment of treatability. The flexibility allowed each examiner by the use of play also provides him with a way to assess the child's use of identification or projection, or regression and so forth, and thus allows another evaluation of the child's potential flexibility and responsiveness to help.

As mentioned earlier, the parents are always involved in the evaluation of children and their treatability. The parents are evaluated not only because they help determine the child's psychopathology, or are caught within and themselves disturbed by it, but also because the child depends upon them for his very process of growth. All of us know the crucial part that parents play in a child's concept of himself, of others, and of the world itself. Similarly, the parents' concept of the evaluation process is crucial to the child's concept of it. Rarely in the evaluation or the treatment of adults are others' opinions as vital as they are to the evaluation and treatment of children. As a child goes through his growing up, his parents must have the ability to adjust to each change and be able to modify their view and expectations of him so that these will be appropriate to the developmental change itself. In the evaluation process, the child undergoes an experience which allows the examiners to decide whether they think parents have some ability to adjust to change within the child and, thus, will be able to support changes which hopefully will occur in treatment—changes which cannot be maintained without their support.

The team must always weigh the fact that a child is *brought* to therapy while most adults *seek* therapy. Motivation for help usually comes first from parents or from outside the home and, therefore, external threats are always involved in it. It is always necessary to evaluate the amount of resistance the child will muster when the evaluation process implies a separation from parents. Since the evaluation also implies some dissatisfaction with the child as he is at present, he may view the process as threatening loss of love or rejection by his parents. And since all child referrals are to some degree authoritarian, to this degree the team must deal with the child's resistance to coming to the clinic.

The child's relationship with the examiner, just as later with his therapist, includes both a real and a transference relationship; however, since he and his parents are all vividly participating in the evaluation process, his problem of identifying with the examiners is always likely to involve problems of a real relationship as well as those of a transference relationship.

PITFALLS

Levine (1952) states that two processes are involved in coming to an understanding of dynamic diagnosis through evaluation. He cites the first of these as an intellectual process involving perception, logic, and reason and the second as an empathic process requiring a limited and temporary identification with the patient.

In working with children, the examiner may easily fall into the several dilemmas that Levine poses: namely, sympathizing too much with the patient's attempt to blame others; participating too greatly in his anxiety; agreeing too readily with his viewpoint; taking too strongly permissive an attitude toward his neurotic needs; or expecting too little from the child in the way of performance and adjustment. The examiner must be able to empathize but yet not lose his *own* identity.

In the evaluation process, hopefully, the child and the examiner have a vital responsive relationship but the constant purpose must be the diagnostic study, which is to gain understanding of how the child and the family can be helped to bring about a beneficial change in the child's behavior; this purpose is easily defeated if the examiner needs to satisfy his own neurotic conflicts through the diagnostic relationship with the child. If overidentification leads to the examiner's failure to appreciate the multiple and varying aspects of the roles played by different persons in the child's life, then he fails to achieve a dynamic understanding of the actual complex interplay between the child and others. Friend (1952) points out how easily people may become transformed into fixed images and how quickly the evaluation is led into rigid generalizations and arbitrary concepts that can only lead to falsely evaluating the problem and its treatability.

> *Case Example:* Walter was a peculiar two-and-a-half-year-old, with no speech sounds beyond grunts and extraordinary rigidity of posture, movement, and expression. Interviews with the mother revealed that she had been excessively rigid in her obedience to the pediatrician's early suggestion that she give the baby a suppository if he did not have a bowel movement; this she had continued to do from the child's early infancy to the present, never allowing him to move his bowels voluntarily. This pattern made it difficult for the team to appreciate the many warm qualities and strengths of this mother who had been so overzealous in this regard. The combination of (1) casework help for the mother, (2) eliminating the suppositories, and (3) providing extra support for participating in nursery school activities and communication was rewarded by normal language and behavior by the end of two years of treatment.

When the examiner's overidentification with the child allows him to derive unconscious, vicarious pleasure or anger from the child's problem or when he unconsciously assumes omnipotent attitudes toward the child and the problem, his distorted understanding will result in inappropriate recommendations for treatment. In all these various ways, the evaluation of a child and his family, as well as the subsequent evaluation of the treatability of the child's problem, frequently requires even greater maturity from the team than does the evaluation of adult patients.

The larger complex of relationships which is under scrutiny in the study of a child and his problems means not merely that the parents must always be involved in such an evaluation but that the child must be studied in totality, which includes his specific constitutional and biological equipment, his pattern of growth and development, his individual experiences, and his role in the family and the social group. Each of these variations must be considered individually and in relation to each other, then related to the final diagnosis of treatability

In regard to the variations in constitutional and biological factors, we know, for example, that a specific pattern of brain damage not only creates a handicap to which the child and his parents need adjust but also specific difficulties in the inner adjustive process itself.

> *Case Example:* Barbie, a brain-damaged girl of thirteen, shows increased loss of motor coordination and integration in speech and in thought when under stress of overstimulation, noise, new and complex situations, tests, or such disturbing conditions in the family as conflict, argument, and hostility between other family members. The same is true when she is ridiculed or attacked by peers. Thus, the brain damage not only interferes with specific academic and athletic skills, such as arithmetic or riding a bike, but also seriously interferes with the adaptability required for life in a vigorous family and school situation, as well as with her feeling secure in areas of mastery and adjustment.

In regard to the variation in growth and development, we not only see that the general rate of development varies in different children but that its various aspects do not always proceed at the same rate within the same child.

Case Example: Developmental variation can be seen in Arthur, who is hypersensitive to external stimulation, verbally very bright, but lacking in the muscular vigor to defend himself against other boys. Such a child may realistically retreat or be extremely selective in regard to participation in potentially overstimulating and overdemanding group activities, while enjoying reading, writing, drawing, or music—in any or all of which he may make rapid advances. The discrepancy in developmental levels may appear as intellectual precocity accompanied by social immaturity; this slower rate of social maturing may contribute to greater temporary dependence on his parents and other adults.

Each developmental step a child takes is tentative and he may normally fluctuate from one level of adjustment to another during the transition. In children, we see not only a relative lack of stabilization of the developmental process at certain moments but also this same relative lack of stabilization in the symptoms and the psychopathology. Thus, regression, which we more frequently see in a child than in an adult, carries with it less serious psychopathological significance. It is a mechanism that a child can more easily use since it is more readily available to him, and is a defense mode from which he can more easily return to behavior appropriate to his age than is usually true for adults. As a matter of fact, temporary regressions are a normal aspect of transitions both from the preoedipal period to latency (many an eight-year-old still wants a lap or a shoulder to cuddle against at tired moments) and from latency to adolescence.

Furthermore, direct restitution in therapy is possible to a greater degree in a child than in an adult, a factor which needs to be evaluated in coming to an appraisal of the child's treatability. This is especially true during the preschool years when the child is more fluid, more volatile, and more likely to go to extremes, as well as more quickly able to relinquish disturbing behavior patterns when his inner perceptions are clarified and his feelings and conflicts are relieved. In relation to the variation in individual experience, we need only add in our attempt to understand the evaluative process that any specific etiological factor may contribute to any one symptom or combination of symptoms in different children, and, conversely, any specific form of behavior in a child may result from interaction between a variety of etiological factors.

Finally, in regard to the variation in social modality, Erikson (1963) has helped us realize that there is not only a timetable of drive development related to maturing social functions evoked or expected by society but that there is a timetable of ego development as well.

Our hope is that, in addition to arriving at a historical understanding of a child's problem (why this child needs help), we can also arrive at an understanding of its immediate genesis (why this child needs help *now*). However, a recommendation for treatment is looked upon not merely from the standpoint of relieving the immediate problem but also with the hope of freeing this child for further developmental growth within his family. Out of the immediate evaluative situation, the team learns of the expectations of both the parent and the child and can become aware of those factors which may prove serious barriers to or supports for the later process of help.

Thus, in order to arrive at a diagnostic evaluation which lends itself to the evaluation of the treatability of the child within his total setting, the team needs to understand four major areas:

The dynamics within the child. This includes his constitutional equipment and course of growth; the sequences and interaction of evolving drives and ego development; the defenses he uses; the secondary gains he makes from dealing with his problems; the conflict-free areas of the child's ego functioning and other personal resources; and his current and potential adaptive progress within his social-cultural group.

The dynamics of the parent-child relationship. This includes an evaluation of the parental attitudes and those defenses which the child uses in his interaction with his parents; the degree of conflict between the gratification of the child's desires and that of either or both parents' demands; the ability of the parents to deal with their own feelings and anxieties about the child and their relationship with him; the ability of the parents to deal with their feelings and anxieties about the potential competition from the therapist-child relationship; the ability of the parents to accept change in the child; and the strengths and assets of the parents as observed in their ways of coping with the interplay of forces in the total current situation between themselves and the child.

The dynamics of the child's adaptation to others outside the family group and his ability to achieve a new relationship with them. This includes the conflict between the child's own desires and of the culture, as well as the useful and the pathological defenses which he has developed in his effort to cope with the social and cultural group. Thus, we need a complete description of the positive as well as the disturbed aspects of the child's behavior at school and in the neighborhood, with adults and with peers.

The probable dynamics of the therapist-child interaction, with an attempt to evaluate the expectable interactions both at a real and transference level. This involves not only a thorough evaluation of the child's behavior and attitudes in several diagnostic sessions, but also an evaluation of the potential therapist's own self-awareness and the effects of his probable attitudes and responses in working with this damaged, destructive, clinging, or depressed child.

In all of the above areas, we ask not only how the child has struggled inwardly and outwardly and with what combination of self-defeating, socially intolerable, and actually or potentially constructive—or even creative—outcomes. We also ask to what extent the child's adaptive patterns are primarily in response to his conflict with a genuinely difficult environment and which ones reflect an already internalized conflict within him. We need to become aware of the meaning of his symptoms, or of his behavior, in terms of the predominant areas of conflict and his probable capacity for effective, satisfying functioning.

We also need to be aware that the course of every child's growth and development into an adult always involves dynamic struggle and conflict. There is conflict between drives, such as between his need both to love and to hate his parents; between ego and drives, especially between the child's longing to keep the satisfactions of childhood while resisting its limitations on his maturation and autonomy. Conflicts may even exist at the ego level, as in the case of the teenager who has to make a choice between two mutually exclusive vocational plans; and conflicts between ego and superego also become acute in adolescence. For example, an inner voice protests that it would be cheating when opportunity offers a way to get the exam answers and guarantee a good grade. Conflict arises in part from the fact that gratification of one set of drives, needs, or wishes is sometimes impossible if another set is also to be gratified. Conflict also arises between a child's demands for gratification and those of other human beings with whom he associates closely, particularly his family; or his demands may conflict with the customs and manners of his social group. The matter of evaluating treatability, then, is never one of determining static facts of disturbance, but, instead, always involves understanding a dynamic process.

This understanding is necessary even for the damaged child or the child with multiple vulnerabilities. Whatever defective or ill-assorted equipment contributes to his difficulties, he is still a dynamic, struggling child—with all the vital needs for satisfying relationships, for love and recognition as an individual; as well as with all of the motor urges, sensory hungers, aggressive impulses, curiosities, and drive to mastery of other children. But his intrinsic deficiencies realistically multiply his frustration, his conflicts with the environment and himself. He needs an even more comprehensive and dynamic understanding than the constitutionally normal child.

Child psychiatry came to this awareness through three clear stages of change in the concept of diagnosis (Crutcher, 1943). The earliest stage was that of gathering history and data, which included a detailed description of early development and a conscious delineation of the child's and the parents' problems. In this stage of diagnosis, the responsibility for the correction of the child's problem was given to a therapist who worked with the inner conflicts of the child, while the mother was helped by a social worker to modify her attitudes and to carry out social changes as recommended by the therapist. At a later stage the child's problem began to be viewed as an element in a larger family pattern of disturbance; thus, the development of the child, who was no longer believed to be an independent entity, was considered part of a process dependent to a large extent upon his *relationship* to his parents. However, at this point in the history of child psychiatry, the focusing of treatment on intrafamily relationships resulted in minimizing the necessary diagnostic evaluation of the child and *his* treatability; in other words, there was a one-sided stressing of the parent-child relationship. At present—the third stage—we use the diagnostic study as both a comprehensive evaluative study and a brief treatment service. Treatability can thus be considered from a total diagnostic appraisal of a troubled and disturbing child interacting with and affected by his family and from an evaluation of their response to the help already provided through the diagnostic process itself.

CHAPTER IV

The Psychologist's Contribution

The psychologist's* diagnostic work with the child has often been contrasted with other diagnostic approaches by focusing on his use of tests. Such a way of thinking emphasizes the tools of the trade, the methods rather than the goals. Emphasiz-

* We express gratitude to our colleagues, Alan J. Lieberman, Verlyn L. Norris, and Mark Rudnick for the use of their vivid examples of the relationship between themselves and the children they tested.

ing the psychologist's use of tests is like characterizing an automobile
mechanic as someone who uses a monkey wrench, or a surgeon as
someone who uses a scalpel. It is difficult to destroy the idea that
tests are instruments that automatically provide answers to diagnostic questions. The psychologist must do more than let his material
speak for itself. He must interpret the patient's responses and give
meaning to them, based on his knowledge and understanding of
personality organization.

What, specifically, is the psychologist's contribution to the
diagnostic examination of the child? Some feel that the so-called
X-ray quality of psychological tests gives an unusual insight to the
content of the child's conflict. Others consider psychological tests
to be particularly valuable in outlining the structure of personality
organization, the layering of defenses, and the description of au-
tonomous functions. Still others stress the value of the background
of the psychologist's training—its emphasis on the normal range
of behavior with which supposedly deviant behavior can be compared. These ways of describing the psychologist's contribution are
probably all correct. Sometimes the psychologist contributes special
understanding about the content of conflict, sometimes about the
organization of the personality structure, sometimes about the process that causes the emergence, disruption, and disappearance of
various behaviors. And sometimes he is able to relate what he sees
to the behavior of the normal child. In a specific case he may
contribute in several or all of these ways.

OBJECTIVITY

Quite frequently it is said that what really captures the
psychologist's unique contribution is the objective way he goes
about gathering and interpreting his data. In this connection, one
thinks most frequently of the numbers with which the psychologist
emerges—numbers that represent the shorthand comparisons of a
child's performance with that of other children. And, indeed, although others' confidence in the psychologist's objectivity may be
greater than warranted, it is relatively appropriate to think of objectivity in the area of so-called intelligence testing. If, however,
objectivity means that more subjective impressions do not enter

into diagnostic formulations and conclusions, then the psychologist must disagree. He must explain that even in obtaining an IQ subjective factors do enter—not only in the way the so-called intelligence quotient is derived but also in the way it is interpreted. Certainly, two identical intelligence quotients may not have at all identical meanings.

> *Case Example:* Tom and Bill both achieve an IQ of 100 on the Wechsler Intelligence Scale for Children. On looking closer, we see that they arrive at this figure via quite different routes. Tom obtains a Verbal Quotient of 125 and a Performance Quotient of 75; Bill's Verbal Quotient is 90 and his Performance Quotient 110. Thus while Tom might go through college quite easily, Bill would in all likelihood have major difficulties there. Further, Bill's Verbal Quotient of 90 is the result of adding vastly discrepant subscores, which range from 4–13. Fred's same Verbal Quotient of 90, on the other hand, is the result of subtest scores which are rather homogeneously distributed and do not deviate from each other by more than one or two points.

These different patterns of ability (resulting in the same *total* scores) will be reflected in dissimilar interests, performance, patterns of relationship, feelings of success and failure, identity structures, plans and expectations for the future, and defensive organizations. Furthermore, many of the meanings and inferences based on such scores are derived from a qualitative analysis and a judgment of *how* the child has worked to organize and produce his responses.

> *Case Example:* Frances indicates that a dog has five legs, that we buy sugar in a hardware store, and that we boil water by pouring it on sand. The examiner must judge whether these flagrantly incorrect responses are the result of (1) poor intelligence, (2) confusion and disorganization, (3) angry resistance, (4) testing of the

examiner's ability to see through and accept teasing, or (5) still other reasons. Depending on the psychologist's judgment of what is going on, he will interpret and handle his interaction with Frances very differently. It is obviously not enough "objectively" to score Frances' responses wrong, since this would tell us very little about her efforts to deal with this type of task.

Once we leave the area of intellectual ability, it becomes even more difficult to ascribe absolute objectivity to the psychologist's findings. It is true that a number of tests (for example, the Rorschach) have highly formalized scoring systems that give the impression of objective accuracy. Yet, we find that there are at least four such major systems, that certain Rorschach responses leave much to individual judgment as far as assigning a score is concerned, that subjective factors of experience, judgment and theoretical conviction do enter into the interpretation of such scores.

TESTING AS INTERVIEW

A testing session with a psychologist can be thought of as a type of interview with the characteristics of repeatability and structure. While we think of most interviews as involving two persons in direct communication, the psychologist's test interview is a mediated one. A third party—the test—modifies the directness of a face-to-face relation.

The repeatability of the psychologist's test interview which tends to be the same each time it is given, is more characteristic of work with adults than children. As a child grows, his abilities change. Tasks which are appropriately administered at age four are no longer appropriate two years later. Not only are intellectual abilities different from one age level to the next, but the testing atmosphere becomes different. A psychologist obviously does not interview or test a three-year-old in the same way as a fifteen-year-old, nor does he interview retarded and gifted fifteen-year-olds in the same way. Nevertheless, he does tend to interview similar types of disturbed children in a rather similar way.

One advantage of being able to repeat interviews with little modification is that it gives the psychologist a baseline for comparison. He can see how one child behaves differently from another when faced with the same situation. He is able to compare the same child's performance at one time with his performance at a future time, and he can evaluate changes that have occurred in the interim.

The psychologist not only has the opportunity of comparing a given test on one child with the same test on another child, but also of comparing an entire *battery* of tests on different children. A test battery may be viewed as one large test, composed of complex parts (just as the Wechsler Intelligence Scale for Children is a complex test composed of various subtests). A battery permits a comparison of an entire *sequence* of interviews, a sequence which is conducted in approximately the same fashion from one time to the next. In a sense, the psychologist tests a process over a period of time. He compares one child's handling of the complex sequence with another child's. In this way he may find, for example, that while one child becomes increasingly organized from one day to the next, another becomes increasingly disorganized.

Case Example: George's behavior during the evaluation reflected a picture of deteriorating control, both within each hour and from one hour to the next. At first, he presented himself as an exceedingly friendly, pleasant boy who was most eager to please and to be correct. As our hours together continued, he became more active and restless, although not as yet destructive. Between tasks which required his presence at the desk, he paced around the room, looked out the window, investigated books and papers, and touched, bounced, and felt different objects. At the same time, however, he was usually able to sit down again when asked. At the beginning of our fourth hour, as I came to call for him, he almost hit me with a snowball intended for another patient. Far from being apologetic, he expressed great glee. During this hour he seemed even more excited. He was hypersensitive to what was going on outside the office, racing to the door or window in response to any unusual noise. While working, he complained of inability to concentrate because the shouts of a small boy in the hall were too distracting. He stated that he had had similar experiecnes at home when he would find himself unable to read, write, or watch TV whenever there was extraneous noise.

When he arrived for his fifth hour, his extreme anger was immediately apparent. He pounded the door to my office and demanded that I open it quickly. Once inside, he slammed the door, kicked chairs and other objects, pounded on the wall, cursed, and stated he would do none of the tests. When I handed him the Story Completion Test, he read it and, with a sneer, tore it up very deliberately. He finished two Sentence Completion items in a very aggressive fashion and then stated he would do no more. He began to climb out the window, and when I contained him, he swore at me, threatened to stab and kill me and to break my arms and legs with judo. He accused me of attacking him and said he was aware that I had hidden microphones in the room, which recorded each word he spoke.

On the last day he asked to see me again. He was able to complete the remaining tests quickly and then asked to play catch with me for half an hour. During this last meeting, he behaved very much as he had when he first came and expressed almost no overt anger or aggression.

A parenthetical comment must be made at this point. Persons who are not psychologists (and sometimes those who are) may at times think of psychological testing as a type of assault on the patient. They feel that the tests are an attack on defenses, an attack which leaves the victim powerless to withstand what they might term an aggressive onslaught. Often they feel that certain children simply cannot be tested because they are too disturbed, too vulnerable. We believe, however, that every child can be tested. Testing, at times, requires great patience, and it requires that the psychologist be sensitive to the vicissitudes of the child's anxieties. So long as he modifies his testing approach in accordance with the situation, he cannot "damage" the child. It is an interesting phenomenon that, by and large, as the psychologist gains experience with children—and consequently becomes secure with them—the interaction between the individual child and the psychologist becomes less and less problematical, even in the most disturbed cases.

A further characteristic of the psychologist's interview is that it provides a relatively clear-cut, orderly give-and-take, in which both the psychologist and the child have a rather precise idea of what is expected of each. The child knows that he will be expected to define certain words, answer certain questions concerning general information, or attempt to attribute meaning to vague inkblots. This characteristic of tests is usually referred to as *structure*. Although the meaning of some tasks is more equivocal (that is, less structured) than that of others, the child knows that the psychologist will expect him to deal with them in some particular fashion. Although the Rorschach blots may be so unclear as to permit a rather wide range of responses, the child knows that when he finishes with one inkblot, another will take its place. In other words, a testing session has a regularity about it—the child knows that he will spend the hour essentially in attempting to perform tasks which the psychologist will set for him.

The quality of structure often has important ramifications. Occasionally, a child seems very different with the psychiatrist from what he seems with the psychologist. Often the difference is so great that both of them have the impression of dealing with different children. This difference may come about because the child is much more at ease when his behavior is organized for him, as in the psychological examination; or it may come about because the child feels threatened when organization is imposed. Depending on how he feels when his freedom to take the initiative is limited, the child may show more defensive, anxious behavior to the psychiatrist than to the psychologist. At other times, the situation is reversed. For example, certain mentally retarded children need to exert immense efforts to deny their inability. When they are put in a situation where they must demonstrate what they can do (for example, on an intelligence test), they may become intensely frightened. Their hyperactivity and destructiveness help them to avoid exposing vulnerability and helplessness. If, on the other hand, they themselves can organize their activity, they are better able to disguise their limitations, so that they do not become anxious to nearly the same extent.

> *Case Example:* It was known that Jerry, age ten, was capable of functioning on only a limited basis. For this reason, the psychologist first planned to start testing him at the six-year level on the Stanford Binet. It later became evident that Jerry was able to function at only about a three-year level. The following is an excerpt of a portion of an hour the psychologist spent with Jerry, before he knew that the boy was a much more limited child than he first appeared. Evident here are Jerry's violent efforts to avoid a situation in which his inadequacies would become apparent, both to himself and to the examiner.
>
> "Jerry came to my office, and I started with a Verbal Stanford-Binet subtest. He did not look at what I was showing him. Instead, he looked past me and smiled. I tried to capture his attention, and, laughing and giggling, he began to thow things. He ripped my jacket off its hook and threw several test items to the floor, and he continued to laugh and giggle. He started to rip open my desk and file drawers and to spill their contents on the floor. I took him outside, since I could no longer contain him in the office. There he ran away and picked up objects and tried to hit me with them. He asked me to let him go, saying that he promised he would be good. When I did let him go, he ran to where some toys were stacked and threw these on the ground. During the rest of the hour, whenever I did not physically restrain him, he attempted to hit me with sticks and stones, hurling them at me with all his strength, laughing all the time.

Only when I suggested that we play ball was he able to compose himself again and to become sufficiently organized to play with me in a fairly adequate fashion."

In order to determine if Jerry was capable of behaving differently, he was seen by another psychologist who gave him some very simple nonverbal tasks to do. These were on a two- to two-and-a-half-year level. During these sessions, Jerry displayed none of the excitement and destructiveness that he had shown before. Although he made frequent protests about his inability to perform adequately, he made no serious efforts to avoid the tasks. At times he triumphantly announced the successful completion (to him) of a task; at times he sang to himself while working. Significantly, when the other psychologist asked Jerry to respond to verbal material, Jerry again began to be aggressive and hyperactive. He was so afraid of exposing his lack of ability that he resorted to acting as though he were a "bad boy," who did not do what he was supposed to do because he did not feel like it. As soon as he was given tasks he could handle, he became completely cooperative. He preferred to be thought of as a child who did not want to, rather than as one who could not.

There are children who require leadership from another person. They are unable to map a course of behavior, and they feel helpless when they have to make their own decisions. When it is left up to them what to do, they may retreat into silent inactivity. When these children are brought into a situation such as psychological testing they flourish. They are relieved to be told what is expected of them, and they do what they can in order to please.

OTHER TEAM MEMBERS

It is difficult to conceptualize the difference between what the psychologist obtains from the Rorschach or Thematic Apperception Test and what the psychiatrist obtains from his interview. In fact, sometimes the psychologist and psychiatrist may obtain much the same information from their separate investigations. Other times, the psychologist, through his particular investigation, and the psychiatrist, through his, will emerge with material which is far from identical. Frequently, the findings of the psychiatrist and psychologist supplement one another, but occasionally they are so different that the data seem to conflict and a major integrative effort is required.

If a psychiatrist and psychologist work together productively, they discover that, although each contributes to the understanding of the other, it is almost impossible to distinguish in advance the specific contribution each will make, particularly since it is likely to differ in each instance. Working together productively means communicating freely, noncompetitively and nondefensively.

It is a truism to say that the various team members need one another in order to reach a useful solution to diagnostic problems. When the psychologist discovers something in his testing, he may well wish to discuss with the social worker the background of a particular trait or characteristic in the home situation. Such a brief discussion helps to clarify matters for both parties. If the psychologist finds that the child behaves with him in a certain way, he will wish to check whether the psychiatrist's experiences are similar. These checks will help the psychologist to formulate his own conceptions, and they will result in a much more differentiated final picture of the child.

Case Example: Prior to seeing Sam, who is twelve years old, for the first time, I was informed by Dr. L., the psychiatrist on the case, that Sam was very difficult to reach. He answered questions only with yes and no and was otherwise uncommunicative. Dr. L. wondered whether Sam might be retarded, because he was so unable to speak spontaneously, to be reflective, or to answer with more than his meager "I don't know." Following my first testing session, I gave Dr. L. my impressions according to test results, that Sam was not retarded and his "I don't know" was a defensive operation, used because he did not wish to take a chance on giving a wrong answer or because he wanted to avoid involving himself. I used the example of Sam's being able to name the four seasons of the year after he initially had replied, "I don't know." I asked him to name the present season, the one that followed, and so on; eventually he was able to name them all.

Dr. L. told me the next day that he had interpreted Sam's "I don't know" as a way of defending himself. This interpretation produced extreme anger in Sam, a reaction which seemed to confirm his need to avoid involvement of his feelings and thoughts by using ignorance as a defense.

Although Sam became hyperactive and restless with me whenever he was asked to do something which demanded self-revelatory responses (such as making up TAT stories), he never became angry. Dr. L. and I were thus able to understand the course of Sam's anxiety build-up: When he is asked to deal with a well-structured, emotionally neutral task, he tends to use his defensive ignorance; when the task involves small reflection, as on the projective material, he becomes hyperactive; finally, under direct probing of feelings, he becomes panicky and enraged.

I was, thus, able to tell both the psychiatrist and social worker that Sam was able to function intellectually well within the average range, although he had come with a history of school failure and with a provisional diagnosis of mild mental retardation.

Certain of Sam's attitudes and feelings toward his parents, particularly his mother (feeling that she was neglectful and unavailable; wishing to exchange her for someone else; finding the relationship with her sexually tempting; experiencing guilt toward her), fell into place when the social worker informed me a few days after the beginning of the evaluation that the mother was a severe drug addict who found it impossible, because of her illness, to be an adequate mother and wife. Knowing this,

Sam's projective responses began to make more sense, and I could tell both the social worker and the psychiatrist what Sam's unconscious, preconscious and suppressed reaction to his home situation was. This was particularly useful because, in order to protect his mother, Sam had felt it necessary consciously to dissimulate about the state of affairs at home. Until the information emerged in casework, he constantly had to affirm that things at home were "just fine"; even after his mother had told us about her illness, Sam still needed to protect her by denying that he had bad feeling of any sort toward her.

As this example shows, communication between team members is a continuous process; each fact from another discipline helps in mapping out the examination, since it modifies the approach to the material. The new conclusions which result are communicated in turn, thus leading again to new facts and conclusions—and so the process continues. From team members conveying their impressions to each other and then making use of these, a "truer," more comprehensive, and more useful picture of the patient and the family emerges. The social worker understands the parents' statements and is therefore able to convey more significant information to them. The entire team is in a better position to make recommendations which take into consideration the complexities of the family's situation.

This emphasis on sharing information leads us to a point of view about which, in the past, opinion was widely divided. Should the psychologist make use of previous information, which, for example, may be available from the social worker, or should he, instead, approach the case without prior knowledge? There was a time in the history of psychological testing when the psychologist needed to demonstrate that he could find out what was going on with his tools alone, without help from anyone. Frequently, such activity became a *tour de force*. Thus, after an inclusive battery of tests, the psychologist might demonstrate that the patient seemed overly preoccupied with topics involving fire. Had he looked at the case history, or asked the social worker, he would have discovered that one of the parents' initial complaints was that their child was a fire-setter. In such cases the psychologist demonstrated that, although his instruments and insights were sensitive, his findings were not particularly useful in adding information or understanding to what was already known.

Nowadays, since psychological testing is much more accepted, it is no longer necessary for the psychologist to prove himself and his tools in this way (that is, "scientific"). Rather, the psychologist's findings are of greatest value when they supplement and amplify or contribute to the precision of an understanding which is, a least partially, present from the beginning. In other words, he is not so much concerned with discovering that the patient is a fire-setter as he is with the background of needs (for example, the nature and quality of the patient's wishes and drives, defenses and adaptations, and anxieties and guilts) which cause the child to choose this particular behavior to express his conflict.

TEST ADMINISTRATION

A major characteristic of a psychologist's work with children must be flexibility. He must be sensitive to the child's need to accept, reject, or otherwise modify the way in which the examiner wishes to go about his business. Thus, the psychologist working with a child, in order to achieve best test results, will not be too insistent that the testing be carried out in a certain way. The child is so often made anxious by testing that the testing may become disrupted unless the psychologist flexibly deals with the manifestations of the child's disturbance. It is almost impossible to say in advance what form this flexibility should take. At any rate, the examiner should strive for an elastic attitude and accept (within limits, of course) certain conditions which the child sets. Some examples may indicate the kind of elasticity required:

If a child is afraid of losing control because he sees himself as passive and helpless whenever he is called upon to perform certain tasks, he may insist on reversing roles (such as, sitting in the examiner's chair and asking the examiner questions). If the psychologist is willing to accept such changes in procedure, he will probably find that after a while the child no longer feels so threatened. The child does not feel that the examiner is out to conquer him, and after a while both are able to proceed with testing in the more usual fashion.

Sometimes a child is so fearful and withdrawn that he is able to do tasks only while sitting under or behind some piece of furniture. Here the psychologist must not be too concerned with his dignity.

Sometimes a child is so frightened of being in a new situation in which he is asked questions by a stranger in a strange room that he sits terrified, unable to respond at all. At such times—depending on the relationship the child has with his mother or father —it may be valuable to invite one of them to sit in with the child and have them ask those test questions that he will not answer for the psychologist. This last situation, of course, at times creates new and difficult problems. For example, a mother may be so eager to have her child do well that she finds it difficult to sit quietly when her services are not needed. She may urge the child on to greater productivity or tell the psychologist (in front of the child) that her child can really do all these things at home; in general, she may intrude in such a way that testing becomes considerably more difficult. At such times the psychologist is put on his mettle to temper firmness with courtesy and understanding.

FLEXIBILITY AND STANDARDIZATION

Sometimes the need for flexibility appears to violate the rules for standardized administration that are established to insure reliable and valid test results. Psychologists learn that, in order to have maximum repeatability, they must not only consistently offer the same material but also administer it in identical ways. But to what extent is it desirable or useful to insist on this approach? Is a patient who approaches a test angrily exposed to the same testing situation as one who is relatively contented, simply because both look at, or touch, the same materials? Efforts to enlist the patient's greatest cooperation (even if this means, at times, a modification of the rules of administration) may result in greater reliability, not to say validity, than when the psychologist adheres to standardized procedures regardless of the patient's mood, attitude toward testing, emotional maturity, and ability to handle the test.

> *Case Example:* John is an obedient, "good" boy who is eager to please and who goes out of his way to be co-operative and to show his willingness to abide by the rules of the test. Fred, on the other hand, expresses his fearful-ness of tests through belligerent, belittling behavior. Thus, he attempts to convey that the psychologist cannot overpower him and cannot make him do anything he does not want to do. He attempts to make the intelligence test a battleground. He responds to questions with silence, sarcasm, and silly answers. The psychologist approaches Fred differently from John. Perhaps he wishes only to change the sequence in which he administers the sub-tests. Thus, he may wish to start by letting Fred do things with his hands, rather than talk. John may require occasional praise to do his best; for Fred, praise might be anathema. Encouragement with an answer might help John but only drive Fred further into a sullen resistance. If the psychologist does not adapt himself differently to John and Fred, he may find Fred to be untestable. In order to maintain scientific rigor the psychologist discovers he does so at the expense of not being able to find out what Fred can do.

While we could say that both John and Fred have been exposed to the same stimulus material, we could not say that both had been exposed to the same situation. John sees the psychologist as a person to please, cooperate with, and to impress with his obedience. Fred, on the other hand, sees him as a person who makes unreasonable demands, and tries to make him show up his weaknesses—therefore, someone whom he must defeat.

Of course, whenever the psychologist does change the ad-ministration procedure of a test, he must keep this modification in mind when he interprets his findings. A Rorschach given literally on the run, as a child flits back and forth in the room, can certainly not be interpreted in the same way as a Rorschach administered in a more orthodox way. Still, some kind of test results are a good deal better than none at all; the test is at least a relatively structured situation which affords data on the child's behavior compared to other children in that situation.

Often it is not enough to gain support at the beginning and then rest satisfied. Rapport is frequently gained and lost, and gained again and lost again as the test interview progresses. Particiularly with children it is frequently not enough to establish a good relation at the beginning of the hour, with the hope that this will carry through the entire hour interview. Perhaps as Fred, in the last example, again becomes overwhelmed by the difficulty of the tasks and feels he is being belittled and humiliated, the psychologist will have to modify the technique of administration and even, on occasion, the form of the question. He may wish to give particular support to Fred on questions that he knows will be difficult for him; he may change the stimulus material in order to create a situation that will encourage Fred to do his best and result in the clearest possible picture of the boy's modes of functioning.

Each psychologist has his own idea of what is a valid test situation. Testing involves an interaction filled with meanings for both parties—meanings related to such factors as the patient's need to please or displease, to do well or poorly, to request or reject help, to appear sick or well, or to be dependent or rebellious. While it is undoubtedly true that a modified test loses its accuracy, it is equally true that a test which is not modified to allow for the patient's problems may fail to measure what the psychologist wishes to measure.

Of course, the psychologist must have decided beforehand precisely what it is that he wishes to measure. If, for example, he wishes to see to what degree Fred's anxiety and anger interfere with his optimal performance, then he will not want to change the administration at all. If, however, he wishes to see what strengths and abilities Fred has when his emotional difficulties interfere least with his abilities (that is, if treatment works) and what his capacities and crippling limitations are even when the testing situation is least threatening, then he will need to modify the test administration in such a way as to obtain the richest possible protocol from Fred.

Test administration has to be particularly flexible with children who may seem unstable.

> *Case Example:* Henry was never able to sit at my desk; as he spoke, he often raced from one side of the room to the other. At times he sat far away from me in one of the easy chairs. Occasionally, he lay on the floor or under the table. When it was necessary to work with material at the desk, he came over, did what was required, and then quickly withdrew again. He kept up a constant flow of conversation and only rarely permitted me to speak. His persistent negativism made the outlook for successful testing dim, until it was possible to find the key to exploit it. Thus, on the Rorschach, I was able to obtain responses by asking what the blot did *not* look like. For example, on Card III, he stated, "They don't look like two people at all." He went through all the inkblots, telling me what they did not look like. In this way, with his racing back and forth, retreating under the furniture, and jabbering away, we were able to work our way through the entire Rorschach test. Various modifications of this technique made it possible to have similar success with various other procedures. With a child such as Henry, it is obviously of no use to try test administration in the standardized manner. Henry's terror made it imperative that the psychologist respond flexibly in order to avoid making the relationship into a power struggle which neither party can truly win in any case.

The following exemplifies even more dramatically the need to be flexible and inventive with a child who is frightened of being tested.

> *Case Example:* Chris immediately took command when

we were introduced. He greeted me with enthusiasm, took my hand, and led me out of the waiting room, announcing that he liked Kansas and that he would probably move here. On entering the office, he seated himself in my chair and began issuing orders for me to carry out. For thirty minutes he issued orders, while I made comments about how much safer he felt in a new place with a new person if he were the boss. My shifting to a firm insistence that it was time for us to begin the things that I had planned evoked great anger, threats to have me thrown out, and attempts to bite me when I moved him to his chair. He dissolved into tears, saying that he wanted to be boss and I would not let him; he hoped I felt good! He wanted to move to a different office of his own; then, angrily and threateningly, he created his office within mine, with his own table and chair and all the equipment from my desk. He had another table and chair for his secretary. He ordered me to sit at my desk and work, and to speak only if he gave me "commission" to do so, with many reminders that he was the boss.

When I continued to accept this arrangement in the second hour and suggested that we could take turns presenting work to be done, he became more friendly but kept me silent by telling stories throughout the hour, which demonstrated his strength, resourcefulness, and fearlessness. In the third hour, he showed me an empty office which he had commandeered for his own. He refused to join me in "our" offices upstairs but ordered me to go up and call him on the phone. My phone call, telling him of all the work in the office and of the number of people wanting to know where the boss was, only elicited the order to send the people down to his office. My telling him that I would work at my desk and wait for him to come up brought him into the office in about five minutes, but only to sweep up the equipment from "his" desk and announce that he was moving out. I eventually went to his new downstairs office with some

Children's Apperception Test cards and the request from
a newspaper reporter to the boss that he give stories to
go with the pictures for the newspaper. He eventually
condescended to grant this favor to the newsman and
over the next several hours produced some eight stories.
It was gradually possible to omit the newspaper man and
even to insert a few verbal subtests from the Wechsler
Intelligence Scale for Children. His proprietary interest in
"his" office relaxed slightly, also.

In the seventh hour, he showed me the cigarettes
that he had smoked with the psychiatrist, and he demanded that I give him one also, assuring me that he
often smoked at home. He showed me how well he could
smoke, assured me that cigarettes were good for nine-year-
old boys and helped them to grow big. He initially pro-
tested, but then accepted, my refusal to give him a cigarette because they sometimes made people sick, even
nine-year-olds, and I wouldn't want him to be sick. He remained quite friendly during that hour, and he was more
cooperative than he had been at any other time. In the last
hour, however, when I again refused him a cigarette, he
developed another tantrum, and a repetition of the first
hour followed, although this was now much less intense.
He became very angry, pacing the floor and muttering
threats. He ordered me out of the office at gun point; he
took away all test materials, promising that I would never
see them again. He then shifted to cajolery, saying, "My
dad 'trusts' you. Come on, give me a cigarette!" He tried
pleading, "Just one, just for me. I'll never ask again,
cross my heart." Then he resorted to bribery: "If you
give me a cigarette, I'll stop being like this." He then
reverted back to threats, indicating that he would hang
me and take all of my cigarettes after I was dead. Finally,
he ordered that I give him bubble gum, which I did.
After some further castigating remarks, he was spontaneously able to return a test booklet which he had
previously taken from me. He was again friendly, al-

though he would do little in the way of testing. He spent most of the time demonstrating "dangerous tricks" which he could do (fearfully and awkwardly), such as walking on a ledge in the room or climbing on top of the file cabinet. He pointed out several times that if he was this smart and daring, I would soon know that he should be boss and also that he did not need to go to school.

In addition to flexibility—and related to it—is the need for considerably more *spontaneity* and *informality* with children than with adults. There should be more of a gamelike quality about the interaction, particularly with very little children. At the same time, it is important to avoid conveying to the child that he is going to play games with the psychologist. Tests are not games, and the child knows it. If he is told ahead of time that he is going to play games, the psychologist will find that, while the child is attempting to solve certain items on the Stanford-Binet or Merrill-Palmer, his eyes surreptitiously (and sometimes not so surreptitiously) search the room in order to find where the games are hidden. Although tasks which we ask very young children to do may appear gamelike to the adult, they often are difficult for the child, who may or may not find them fun.

While the psychologist must avoid giving the child (particularly one who is hyperactive and difficult to restrain) the impression that there are no limits to what he may do in the testing session, it is advisable, particularly with younger children, to decrease the emphasis on the businesslike character of the testing. Thus, the psychologist takes time out to listen to the child's story of what he has done just before coming to the clinic; off and on, he lets the child play with various objects to help diminish tension. He does not talk with a five-year-old as though he were an eighteen-year-old —or vice versa.

Case Example: Phyllis, age five, tends to relate very much on a question-and-answer basis. Many times during our sessions, she asked me where my home was. When I told her that I lived nearby, she told me that she did, too, and that she would be able to come over frequently to play with me. It became evident that Phyllis was not at all interested in the content of my responses; rather, she used questioning as a way of establishing and maintaining a relationship. On the Rorschach and Children's Apperception Test, she typically responded to each card by asking what it was. When I, in turn, asked her, she invariably told me what it looked like to her.

Phyllis felt quite free to express her wishes, usually quite directly. She told me what she would like to do or not do. When she had enough of a particular task, she said "I'm froo," in no uncertain terms. But she was able to continue if asked to do so. She was never destructive or hyperactive, and her play never went out of bounds. Aggression was expressed teasingly and always with a smile. When, for example, I exerted a little more pressure than she could handle comfortably, she said, "You rascal" or "You little stinker" and squeezed my finger with her nails.

The child's relatively underdeveloped capacity to handle tension for any extended period of time has important testing implications. It is rarely wise to test a child for more than one hour at a time. He usually is unable to manage a longer time without becoming bored, restless, tired, and generally unhappy. The younger the child, the shorter the testing time should be. Thus, with an infant, it is desirable to arrange frequent and short rest periods, even during the brief overall period of testing. At these rest times the child can sit, lie, or lean back and gather strength for another brief testing period. The three- or four-year-old child rarely maintains interest in testing for more than half an hour or forty minutes. On the whole, the younger the child, the more desirable it is to have frequent play breaks. For example, a child may urge that he be given permission to take time out to play with a toy truck. A good way to deal with such requests is to effect a compromise. The psychologist may suggest to the child that perhaps he can do one or two more tasks, then play for a little while before returning to the test again. Most children will accept such a compromise.

Case Example: Harry was a three-year-old boy with speech problems. I had Pegboard A ready for him, but he barely looked at it. He sat, quietly sucking on a balloon, and holding a toy car in one hand. I brought out a xylophone and Harry's face lit up. He then brought out another xylophone, a large Nest of Cubes, and an extra Seguin Form Board. He gave me one of the xylophones, and I started to play on it. He watched me, sucked on his balloon, and held his ear.

After a little while, on his own initiative, he began correctly to place the blocks of the Seguin Form Board. After he had done this twice, he took the Nest of Cubes and attempted to fit them into the Seguin spaces. Then he tried to put the larger cubes inside the smaller ones. He was finally able to fit all the cubes except one, and he indicated that he wanted me to help him. I did help and told him that I had another Nest of Cubes. When I offered the Merrill-Palmer Set to him, however, he showed no interest whatsoever.

He went to the cupboard again and took out some playing cards. He indicated, without words, that he wanted the table cleared and began to take some of the items off the table himself. He threw the cards to me one at a time, and I placed them in rows. This went on for some time. Then I asked him where I should put a card, and he motioned where I should place it.

I presented him with Pegboard A again and drew his attention to it. This time he became interested and completed it twice. When I presented it a third time, however, he became interested in the xylophone and played it instead. He also gave me one to play. After he had played a while, he returned to the pegboard. Finishing with this, he ate a cookie that I had given him. I then presented Pegboard B, and he completed it quickly. He took the pegs out and used one of them to play on the xylophone. He gave me the other xylophone to play and resumed fitting pegs into Pegboard B.

After he had done this, he again cleared off the table, picked up a ball, and began to roll it back and forth to me. We did this for some time, and he obviously enjoyed himself. I then took out the blocks, and he spontaneously built a tower ten blocks high. It fell down, and, undismayed, he started a new one. This he built twelve blocks high, and it also fell down. I showed him how to make a Three Cube Pyramid, and he very quickly copied what I had done. He began to make several Three Cube Pyramids on his own and then made a long row of blocks on top of which he placed another. He pushed his train to the edge of the table and began to push it off the end. When I held my hand there, he smiled and started pushing the train in the other direction. When I indicated to him that he should put all the blocks back in the box, he did this very readily (in this way completing another Merrill-Palmer subtest).

All in all, we were able to do a great deal by alternating between what he wished to do and I wished to do. At times I would suggest that we do something, and then he would propose an activity. Then I again asked him to do something that I had in mind, and in this way we made considerable progress.

It is sometimes difficult for the psychologist to discover how far he can go with permissiveness. If he is too easy going, the child may be anxious to find out what the limits of permission are. If the psychologist has strong conflicts about permissiveness, he may find that his sessions with the child become chaotic. The child may refuse to be tested, and the psychologist may need all his energies to keep him from destroying test material and office equipment. The psychologist may even have to prevent the child from physically attacking him or himself.

Because very young children have difficulty staying with any one task for an extended period of time, most tests for them are constructed to include a wide variety of things to do. The tests of the Merrill-Palmer Scale, for example, are quickly done and involve great variety. But the psychologist must do more than rely solely on the structure of the tests. He has to take immediate advantage of the child's shifting interests. For example, if while doing the Seguin Form Board the child suddenly picks up a pencil and starts drawing, it is a good idea to take advantage of this momentary interest and to encourage the child to draw or write not only what he wants but also to copy circles, crosses, or stars, as is required in another portion of the test.

It is usually undesirable to have many items available to the child at any one time. He becomes perceptually overwhelmed and may go haphazardly from one thing to another, without being able to involve himself in any particular one. For this reason, especially with a hyperactive child, it is often not wise to permit him to choose the next test item (for example, on the Merrill-Palmer, where it is suggested that he do so). Emotionally disturbed children have a tendency to take one box, open it and discard it, go to another box, open it and discard it, and so on. The psychologist might make it clear at the beginning that *he* will provide the next task once the old one has been completed.

In general, overstimulation can be minimized by having the testing room quiet and free from distractions. It is desirable, as far as the testing area is concerned, to have an arrangement which allows sufficient space for an active child not to feel hemmed in and also permits the setting up of additional equipment; at the same time, the space should not be so large that the child is tempted to run away from the testing place in order to investigate far corners of the room.

Just as the psychologist must take immediate advantage of the child's shifting interest, so must he be aware of the child's shifting levels of ability from one day to the next. The child, more than the adult, is likely to be influenced by such external factors as fatigue, mood, the time of day, and the preceding activity. The examiner frequently finds, therefore, that if a child cannot do a particular task one day, he can often complete it satisfactorily the next. When he has doubts about the child's ability in a certain direction, he may find it extremely valuable to redo an item or even a number of items. Sometimes the readministration of the Rorschach Test gives a different picture from one day to the next. The child has not yet internalized many of the traits of character, personality, and ability that will become part of him later on. Since he is still greatly influenced by the external things of the moment and subject to change as the environment changes, he is more variable in his performances, not only from day to day but even from moment to moment.

> *Case Example:* George, a three-year-old, was tested while in nursery school. Just before the examiner showed him Card V of the Rorschach, George went to the window to look at the other nursery school children, whom he had heard playing outside. After some discussion about playing with friends, the examiner presented Card V. George said "Debbie." On inquiry, it turned out that Debbie was George's favorite friend, whom he had seen climbing on the jungle gym when he looked out the window.

A child is usually more affected by failure than is the adult. For this reason the psychologist should start at a level where he feels quite certain the child will pass. If he does not, the child may react by withdrawing, by becoming negativistic, or by becoming hyperactive and destructive. Nor should the psychologist leave the child with a feeling of failure. Thus, he may wish to provide pleasant experiences at the end of a testing session. Some psychologists arrange the testing session so that failures are interspersed with successes. Here again the examiner must choose between obeying the precise rules of administration and modifying procedures somewhat in order to achieve more useful results in a given case.

In this connection the role of rewards comes up. If the examiner can overcome equating rewards with bribes, he will feel free to discover that a child usually reacts with real pleasure to being given either verbal or more concrete rewards. Generally, a reward gives the child added impetus to continue. Some children constantly ask for rewards in the form of praise, and then it is usually better to discuss this need with them. Nor is it ever good to tell a child he is doing well when he is not; he usually sees through this. Although complimenting him when he does well is quite appropriate and usually appreciated, it often is more effective to give something more tangible, such as a candy or cookie, to a very young child, who does not yet understand the symbolic value of verbal rewards.

Some, however, may raise the objection that by gratifying oral needs, the psychologist encourages regression. But under certain circumstances this is desirable. As the child finds himself face to face with difficult tasks or with failures, he quite likely needs to regress. When he is permitted periodically to act much younger, he is often able to return with new vigor to his appropriate age level and to solve problems that he could not before. Regression represents a kind of safety valve for the child, just as do periods of play and rest. As in all things, of course, moderation must be observed. The child should be helped not to rely on total, chronic regression. His need to regress and his capacity to return to behavior adequate for his age are themselves important diagnostic data.

On the first day of testing, when the child faces the problem of going to a new place with a new person, the psychologist should not overwhelm him with his strangeness. Except for leading the way to the office, the psychologist usually does well to wait until the child comes to him, both physically and psychologically. In extreme cases, particularly with autistic children, it works best when the psychologist removes himself as far as possible and lets the child gradually approach from his refuge. The psychologist might take out a toy or simple test task and play or work with it, ostensibly paying little or no attention to the child. Gradually, the child—his fear somewhat abated and his curiosity somewhat aroused—may come nearer and nearer to see what is going on. This may not happen during the first session, but perhaps during the second, or third, or fourth.

During the first several sessions, the child with a separation problem will be concerned about his parents. If he becomes markedly anxious, the psychologist may wish to show him where his parents are. Even if they are in conference, it may be wise briefly to interrupt, so the child can say hello to his family. Sometimes, as suggested, the only way in which the psychologist can examine a child is not to separate him from his parents at all. He may invite the child's mother or father to sit in briefly during the testing. Sometimes the parents must attend each testing session for the entire time; sometimes the child feels sufficiently secure for them to leave within a few minutes after the initial session begins.

> *Case Example:* Carl was sitting sadly on a chair in the receptionist's office when I first was introduced to him. He did not respond to my greeting, and when I asked whether he would like to come upstairs with me, he looked straight ahead and shook his head. Nevertheless, he did come with me, clutching a ball in one hand and a toy panda in the other. As I closed the door to my office, he suddenly became quite anxious and indicated that he wished to leave. I asked whether he would like to see his parents and he nodded vigorously. Once he saw his mother in the social worker's office, he buried his face in her lap, responding neither to his father nor to anyone else in the room. Accompanied by his parents, he returned to my office; he stood near the door, unwilling to touch the form board that I had set out. I offered various toys from my cupboard but Carl remained shyly withdrawn. Suddenly his eyes caught something which interested him, and going swiftly to the toy cabinet, he returned with the Seguin Form Board. Enthusiastically he proceeded to place the various forms, quite oblivious to the fact that his parents were saying good-bye to him. He was able to stay with me for the rest of the hour without difficulty.
>
> The separation anxiety noted this first hour recurred several times thereafter. Once, when I frustrated Carl by not permitting him to open the Merrill-Palmer suitcase, he suddenly ran to the door and could not be comforted until I took him to see his mother. Another time

his mother was not downstairs when we finished. Carl looked for her in the waiting room; then he pointed outside, obviously hoping that she would be there. We went outside, and I explained to him that his mother would return soon. But Carl's expression suddenly changed into one of intense grief, and he broke into inconsolable sobs. Once reunited with his mother, Carl totally ignored me. Interestingly, each time he left my office, he needed to take something of mine with him—a doll, some beads, or something of the sort. These were items in which he had displayed little or no interest during the hour, and it was apparent that his taking them reflected no particular fascination with the objects themselves. It seemed, rather, that their significance lay in the fact that they were mine —he wished to maintain the continuity of our relationship in this way.

It frequently helps the child to bring something familiar to the psychologist's office. He can be encouraged to bring a toy with which he has been playing in the waiting room while with his mother. This toy can serve as a transition between what is familiar and what is not yet familiar. During the second or third session, the psychologist can have a familiar object from preceding sessions waiting for the child.

Even a quite normal child may feel uncomfortable when he meets a new adult, who, naturally, is so much taller than he. For this reason, and particularly with very small children, it is wise to have a set of small testing furniture available. In this way the psychologist can literally come down to the child's level. Sometimes, of course, a growing child resents being relegated to a "little-baby" position and prefers to sit at the examiner's desk. When the psychologist is in doubt, he may wish to have both the smaller and larger furniture available and to ask the child where he would prefer to work.

There are a number of reasons why it is desirable to test a child over an extended period of time. Seeing a child for six to eight hours over several days (more or less, as seems appropriate) makes it possible for him to open up gradually. He feels more at ease to express himself as he truly feels, and he does not tend to be so inhibited by the pressures of time and strangeness. It is interesting and important for the psychologist to see how a child develops over a period of several days. He can observe nuances of change (and differences which may be much more than nuances) as the child feels more familiar with him. Many children, for example, need to put their best (or worst) foot forward, an attitude which they are well able to maintain if the test interview lasts for only one or two hours. However, they find it much more difficult—and often much less necessary—to continue trying to make some kind of impression over a longer period of time. As time passes, some children become more organized, others less so. The psychologist is much more likely to see the kaleidoscopic range of a child's behavior when he has sufficient time in which to observe it.

> *Case Example:* Larry is a mass of paradoxical contradictions. In our first session, his swaggering gait, casual clothes, flaunted cigarette, brusque manner of speaking, and air of cynical toughness all proclaim his utter disinterest and contempt for the examiner and his tests. In our last session, Larry spontaneously mentioned that it was our last meeting, seemed very tense, at times close to tears, and readily admitted that he had enjoyed talking with me and was reluctant to leave.

The psychologist is not at his best under hurried circumstances, either. He needs time: he may wish to check further on certain hypotheses, give additional tests to discover more about areas in which he feels unsure, recheck certain items because he knows a child fluctuates greatly in his ability from one day to the next, and readminister portions or all of a Children's Apperception Test or portions or all of the Arithmetic subtest of the Wechsler Intelligence Scale for Children. Thus, to his observations the psychologist can add the results of more intensive and extensive testing, which permits the child to develop and to show himself in all his complexity.

A few words should be said about the psychologist's use of interpretive statements during testing. In general, we may state the rule of thumb that interpretations should be made to the child only to facilitate testing. The primary purpose of the psychologist's examination is to gain diagnostic information. Whenever the patient's anxiety or anger interferes with this goal (that is, when testing bogs down and the patient is evasive, fearful, sparse in his replies, or refuses to continue altogether), then it is not only desirable but necessary to interpret the patient's difficulty.

Case Example: Following the administration of the first Rorschach card, which came during the third hour of testing, Dan remained aggressively silent and assumed a facade of boredom. He mumbled, yawned, swung around in his chair with his hands thrown over his back, and dropped his head as if he were falling off to sleep. He did not answer any of my questions, and his silence was tantalizing. Except for a rocking motion that he made while sitting, one might have thought that he was truly bored. This rocking motion was at times quite vigorous and might well have been related to the degree of his anxiety. For example, on the Wechsler-Bellevue Intelligence Scale, the rocking increased on items with which Dan was having difficulty; it decreased on those which he found easy. Only after I had explained that I would not participate in a power struggle and left the initiative up to him was he able to continue with the testing. After discovering that a power struggle was pointless, he became a different boy. Although he did not completely relax, he became responsive. He spoke more easily, moved his chair closer to the desk, and readily handled the test materials.

Dan obviously needed to pit his strength against the strength of adults. In one way or another, he constantly acted out his need to declare his independence. While it would have been inappropriate to deal with this conflict in detail during the testing, it was necessary to focus on it in a limited way, so that testing could proceed at all.

Since children do not usually find tests particularly gratifying, they may wish to use periods of "just talking" as a way to escape. By no means should these periods be minimized. Often the psychologist is able to find the answer to a question by asking the patient directly. One sometimes gains the impression that it is not legitimate to gain information except through the complex process of inference. Why this should be so is hard to understand—perhaps it is a feeling that information acquired indirectly is somehow more elegant or "real." Nevertheless, when the psychologist works as a member of a team it is wise to leave therapeutic interpretations to the psychiatrist. Otherwise testing becomes too easily diluted and too drawn out and confusing to the patient. A psychological test examination and a therapeutic interview involve quite different attitudes, for both the patient and the examiner. Any psychologist who later has taken a patient whom he himself has tested into therapy, knows the importance of changing such a patient's set from a passive respondent one to a set involving a willingness and ability to take more active responsibility.

KINDS OF TESTS

Every psychologist finds himself more at home with certain tests than with others. He has favorite tests which, he feels, give him the most useful information. For this reason we cannot make a pronouncement about what tests should ideally be administered to a child. Nevertheless, it may be helpful to state which particular tests or types of test we have found to be most useful at the Menninger Clinic's Children's Service.

In general, we begin with a test whose purpose is to investigate the *cognitive* aspects of functioning. Often—particularly when we are dealing with a retarded or brain-damaged child—we give two intelligence tests (for example, the Stanford-Binet and Merrill-Palmer, or the Stanford-Binet and Wechsler Intelligence Scale for Children).

In this connection, it hardly needs to be said that there is no such thing as "the" IQ. Different tests result in different scores, depending to a large extent on the proportion of verbal or performance tasks involved in each. Much has been said about the value (and lack of it) of the Intelligence Quotient. While at one time this figure was perhaps overvalued, the tendency at the present time seems to go in the opposite direction. Clinicians are prone to say that they are not interested in a figure or in a number but, rather, in a process. While this aim is commendable, it still seems as though a specific, objective figure which represents an abstraction of different skills and abilities is a useful piece of information. It is undoubtedly true that this figure may hide as well as reveal, but the danger of confusion exists only if the number is divorced from the data it reflects.

There can be no doubt that it is useful to know that a child who appears relatively dull is nevertheless able to achieve an Intelligence Quotient of, say, 115. It is similarly important to know that a child who has the facility of sounding bright, alert, and knowledgeable is unable to achieve an IQ higher than, say, 80. The numbers *115* and *80* are a shorthand way of conveying significant information. In order to learn more, one investigates specific responses. The systematic investigation of various intellectual tasks as they are presented on intelligence tests permits an important check of clinical appearance. A child's score on intelligence tests is a gauge of at least one aspect of ego strength.

Although the final IQ abstraction is important, we are particularly interested in the cognitive style with which the child deals with problems. For this reason we find it of utmost value to make a verbatim transcription of the child's every word, every pause, every gesture.

See, for example, how differently five children answer the same question from the Wechsler Intelligence Scale for Children and how much would be lost if the answers, instead of being written down, were just given the scores 2, 1, or 0.

> *Question:* What should you do if you lose one of your friend's dolls?

Answers:

1. Replace it.
2. Then the police would come. Cause if a girl killed her Mommy and Daddy, the police'll come.
3. Buy her— No! Tell her you're sorry. Save money and buy her a new one. If they don't have the same, ask what she wants. What's my mother doing? Let her come in here. It's too long to wait.
4. Well, if I did. You mean on purpose? [!] Well, go tell your friend; look for it, if they can't find it, both save up money and buy a new doll. [Why both save?] Because I lost it, and she was careless to give it to me.
5. I don't know. I don't know. Just go over and tell her. She'll probably get mad at me, and I'll stay at home. Nobody will play with me. Jean is jealous. If I had all the luxuries in the world, it wouldn't satisfy me because I can't decide what to buy. I'm sort of stingy. I don't know what to do with my money, whether to burn it or what.

From this small sample of answers we can see the marked differences which children demonstrate in answering the same questions. Obviously the psychologist finds out much more than whether the child can answer the question correctly.

From the intelligence test, particularly, we are interested in finding out the cognitive style or the detailed pattern of abilities and limitations of the child, his ways of using his capacities, his specific reactions to failure, his ability to use support and help, and his response to success. We learn about experiences which are followed by regressive behavior, experiences which result in improved integration, areas of functioning which are found to be enjoyable or distressing, and areas which stimulate the most sustained effort as compared with those the child avoids because he finds them meaningless and frustrating.

The intelligence tests used most frequently in the Children's Service are the following: the Cattell Intelligence Scale for Infants; the Gesell Developmental Schedules; the Merrill-Palmer Scale of Mental Tests; the Revised Stanford-Binet Test, Forms L, M, and

LM; the Wechsler Intelligence Scale for Children; the Wechsler-Bellevue; and the Wechsler Adult Intelligence Scale. Occasions arise when special types of intelligence tests are required for children who have such disabilities as deafness, muteness, or blindness or, for other reasons, have problems with language usage. Some of these tests include the Leiter International Performance Scale, the Ammon Picture Vocabulary Scale, the Raven Progressive Matrices, and the Hayes Revision of the Stanford-Binet.

Other tests of significance in the cognitive area include the Bender Gestalt Test, which is particularly useful in revealing abilities and lacks in perceptual-motor organization, and the BRL (Bolles, Rosen, and Landes) Sorting Test, which is helpful assessing the level of the child's conceptual ability—the orderliness and clarity of his conceptual thinking in making useful generalizations and categorizations. The child who has reading problems may usefully be tested with the Durrell Analysis of Reading Difficulty. If the psychologist wishes to evaluate the child's school achievement or reading readiness, he can administer one of the school achievement or readiness tests.

While many of the adult projective tests are useful with children (for example, the Rorschach Test, Thematic Apperception Test, Draw-a-Person Test, and Word Association Test), some of the projective tests particularly constructed for the young (for example, the Children's Apperception Test) seem better suited for younger children. It is often useful to give both the Children's and the Thematic Apperception Tests. Frequently, the psychologist finds that (depending on the test administered) he taps different areas of conflict and different mechanisms for handling them. The differences revealed in defensive and other structures are partly related to the amount of psychological distance which each test permits the child.

We have found it useful to construct a Sentence Completion Form for boys and girls. This form includes items reflecting the child's world, among them parents, siblings, school, and free time. We have found that the child often completes these items explicitly in terms of himself. For this reason, the Sentence Completion Test tends to reveal conscious and preconscious feelings and attitudes, in contrast to other projective techniques which reflect less conscious features.

Sometimes the psychologist must create his own tests in addition to using the more or less standardized tests mentioned above. Such is especially the case when he works with children who are unable to respond to the usual test material because of severe cognitive, emotional, or motivational problems. With such children he may find it necessary to use whatever material is at hand. Thus, for example, he may use a toy, a piece of cloth, a musical instrument, an object which makes noise or fits into something else—anything at hand, in short, which may evoke some type of response. With younger children it is useful to have various toys available. The psychologist may have a doll sitting nearby since young boys and girls often enjoy having it watch them perform. From time to time, a child may wish to play with the doll; thus, the psychologist can use the doll to find out about the child's concepts of numbers or of parts of his body. The doll is sometimes helpful for an initial exploration of the child's sexual interests or his defense against these. Again, flexibility cannot be overstressed. Because the tests the psychologist creates for the moment are not standardized, he must use his material intuitively, imaginatively, and creatively in order to obtain some conception of how the child functions.

> *Case Example:* Betty is a seven-year-old who says no words at all and who seems almost totally uninterested in anything which goes on around her. Only one thing consistently gives her pleasure. She especially enjoys the sound that the drawer of the filing cabinet makes when it is opened and closed. This causes her to laugh heartily. Her eyes blink as she anticipates the sound. She helps push the drawer, sometimes putting her hand on mine and sometimes putting her thumb next to mine. Once her thumb was caught slightly. This caused her to draw her hand away rapidly and to strike me. The minor accident did not interfere, however, with her desire to

continue opening and closing the drawer and laughing with real joy while doing so.

As suggested earlier, it is difficult to know beforehand the precise nature of the information with which the psychologist will emerge. It is equally difficult to make hard and fast rules to cover the exact type of information which each type of test will reveal. We usually expect, for example, that the Wechsler Intelligence Scale for Children will reflect the child's capacity to solve certain kinds of intellectual problems, that the Thematic Apperception Test will give us insight into the content of the child's conflicts, and that the Word Association Test will help us understand the nature of the child's associative process. Nevertheless, we are often surprised.

For example, the child may give an altogether unremarkable performance on the Stanford-Binet, suggesting that his thinking is clear, efficient, and appropriate to his age level. But when given the BRL Sorting Test, his concepts may be peculiar, distorted, and vague. Or the child may give a not particularly interesting Rorschach protocol, in which he reveals only that he wishes to reveal as little as possible. Suddenly, however, on the Children's Apperception Test, he may tell remarkably complex, well-differentiated stories that display an unusual freedom and (by contrast at least)' a readiness to be understood. A breakthrough of this type may occur on any test. Sometimes the child reveals more of his conflicts on the so-called intelligence tests than he does on those specifically designed for the purpose. Sometimes the only indication of underlying pathology occurs on one response to the Word Association Test. Surprises, of course, do not occur only in the direction of pathology. Sometimes the psychologist is amazed to discover how well a child handles, for example, the Bender Gestalt Test, when by all previous indications he should have performed very poorly.

Case Example: Amy's examination presented the psychologist with a double surprise. From tests at previous clinics, he had been told that she had a borderline Wechsler Intelligence Scale for Children, intelligence quotient in the neighborhood of 70, and that she had significant brain damage. When, however, Amy was given all the time she required to show herself to the best advantage, she was able to obtain a much better quotient, to everyone's surprise. Her parents particularly were taken aback because they had thought of and had treated Amy as a retarded girl for almost her entire life.

A less dramatic surprise, and one that is frequently observed, is the following:

Case Example: Janet did so well on the Information subtest of the Wechsler Intelligence Scale for Children that she was able to obtain a weighted score of 16. At the age of eleven, she could designate the capital of Greece, give the correct distance between New York and Chicago, tell who discovered the South Pole, and describe the function of a barometer. Using this performance as a standard, the psychologist expected that she would do well on the Comprehension subtest. Actually, however, Janet achieved a weighted score of only 7 here. Although this discrepancy was surprising, it was explainable. The Comprehension questions brought out Janet's pathology—the severe obsessiveness which made it almost impossible for her to make an intellectual commitment and to sort out the relevant from the irrelevant; the loosening of associations which resulted in her forgetting the original question; the problem with impulse control which made her laugh, giggle, leave her chair, and present dramatic sound explosions, and the intrusions of disturbing thoughts, touched off by the content of the questions.

The psychologist omits tests at the risk of missing out on important information. He cannot, of course, go on testing indefinitely, since there is certainly a point of diminishing returns. When time pressures are great, it may seem that he is indulging himself when he gives numerous tests. However, he must make a choice between testing many patients somewhat or a smaller number much more thoroughly. While the psychologist's activity depends on the point of view of the agency or the clinic in which he works, he has an obligation to convey to others the conditions under which he works most productively and most validly. It is possible to do untold harm if, because of time pressures, an examiner comes to the conclusion that a child is of borderline or defective intelligence when more testing would reveal that, under other conditions, the youngster is able to function normally or if he concludes that a child is only mildly incapacitated when further testing would reveal significant difficulties in reality testing. Although the psychologist can never hope to find out all there is to know, he can strive toward obtaining as clear and undistorted a picture as possible.

INTERPRETATION OF RESPONSES

As of the behavior of any patient, the adequate interpretation of children's behavior depends on the psychologist's thorough grounding in both normal and abnormal psychological functioning. Not only must the child psychologist have an intimate knowledge of the classical syndromes of adulthood, but, in addition, he must have a knowledge of the more specific disorders of childhood. He must be aware that emotional illness in children is usually not crystallized, as it often seems in adults. It is the rare child of whom one can say definitely that a particular illness is of this or that nature. In childhood, it is unusual to find a stable hierarchy or a unification of symptoms into a specific syndrome, for children are growing and constantly changing.

Interpretation of children's responses depends on the psychologist's knowledge of the normal process of maturation. He must have a clear understanding about how and at what particular age part processes and integrative processes become progressively more differentiated. He must know about maturation in the motor sphere, the perceptual sphere, the fantasy and affective spheres, the conceptual sphere, the sphere of causal thinking, and so forth. Further, he must know at what stages of development certain processes emerge which, at another stage, could be considered pathological. Thus, for example, a constricted Rorschach protocol during latency does not have the meanings it might have earlier or later. During latency the child is striving to repress infantile material and is concerned with realistic activity and productivity. Similarly, with an adolescent, the psychologist must be careful to avoid calling all types of inconsistent, stormy, and confused behavior pathological. It is well known that types of thinking and behavior which would reflect a fairly severe disorganization at a later time cannot be viewed with the same degree of concern when they appear in adolescence, since this period is "normally" a stormy time. It is important to remember that, to the degree the psychologist is unfamiliar with age-appropriate behavior, he may interpret characteristics as pathological which actually accord with age-appropriate behavior. In other words, the child psychologist must be familiar with what is typical for each stage through which the child passes in his development. Otherwise he will not be in a position to make a valid statement about the extent of a child's pathology.

What the psychologist interprets and how he goes about it would fill a book itself. However, the following few suggestions may be helpful. Of utmost importance is not only that the psychologist point out the child's areas of difficulty and disintegration but that he describe the areas of strength as well. The child's strengths are foundations on which to build treatment recommendations. The more specifically and concretely the psychologist can spell out these strengths, the more usefully the team can make suggestions for treatment planning.

> *Case Example:* From a prognostic point of view, the outlook for Bruce appears moderately favorable, given the availability of intensive treatment. On the less hopeful side, there is the presence of an unstable identity and a suspicion of others' motives which discourage the formation of a therapeutic relationship. A further complicating factor involves his need to deny that he requires anything from others.
>
> On the other hand, Bruce is able to keep all his evaluation appointments. He can make use of tolerant, good-humored, but firm, relationships and is consistently

able to fulfill all that he is asked to do. He is able to do this despite his tendency to disbelieve that adults can give him the help he needs or that they are on his side. Indications of successful efforts at control, high intelligence, and a developed capacity for self-expression make the outlook for his ability to form a successful therapeutic relationship reasonably optimistic.

How can information be most usefully conveyed to colleagues? The psychologist often finds it difficult to discover the optimal point between, on the one extreme, a presentation of the basic data and, on the other, a presentation of highly abstract and vague speculations, which in their final form produce formulations equally applicable to many people, sick or well, children or adults, male or female. Such formulations, for example, may state "The patient's thinking at times becomes diffuse." Another extreme of equally questionable value is a diagnostic formulation which limits itself to an uninterpreted presentation of what the patient has produced on tests. No effort is made to explain the meaning of the data or to relate them to more inclusive psychological processes. Statements of this type may convey such information as "The patient made dashes instead of dots on the Bender Gestalt Test" or "The patient had four CF responses and only one M response on the Rorschach." While such data are often useful to illustrate more general, abstract inferences, facts must be interpreted in order to have the greatest value. Usually, they do not speak for themselves.

RECORDING FINDINGS

The psychologist must keep in mind that the only goal of his examination is to convey information which he has made as understandable as possible. He must be painfuly aware that the specialized vocabulary of testing, which includes such words as *scatter, syncretism,* and *CF,* means little to people other than psychologists. A report filled with such terms confuses the listener or reader, angers and frustrates him, and, for this reason, often makes the psychologist's contribution less useful.

A report, then, should be written in concise, concrete

language that makes the patient sound human. The psychologist must avoid the pitfall of hyperbole. He should use carefully such words as *always, never, overwhelmingly,* and *extremely.* Indiscriminate use of such adjectives and adverbs makes all psychological phenomena seem alike. If the examiner uses the phrase *overwhelming anxiety* to describe both a child who fidgets uncomfortably in his chair and one who needs to leave the room because of panic he experiences, then the phrase no longer differentiates adequately. Since our language limits the degree to which we can differentiate, it is helpful to give concrete examples; that is, it is useful to tell exactly what the child says and does. In this way the psychologist avoids moribund, empty language, which as a conglomeration of abstractions deprives his description of the child of life and vividness. For the same reason, the psychologist must avoid such common clichés as "The patient is struggling with incestuous wishes toward his mother," "The patient has not resolved his Oedipus complex," or "The patient is suffering from sexual confusion." It is not enough to say that the patient has problems with aggression, or rivalry, or hostility, or anxiety. It is necessary, instead, to understand the situations which produce various reactions in the patient and to trace the development of such processes and the sequences in which one process gives way to another. It is important to know how rivalry, for example, is expressed, what situations give rise to this feeling, and what situations result in its disappearance, attenuation, or intensification.

The psychologist should avoid the pitfall of adhering to what is psychologically fashionable at the moment. For example, it has been fashionable to think of schizophrenic children who do not function at their optimal capacity as having a higher potential. Frequently, one wonders on what basis such a conviction is founded —particularly when the child has been seen only briefly and has not been tested. The examiner must remember that adherence to a particular fashion stands in direct opposition to the psychologist's credo of making a careful examination of the behavior which the child manifests.

Similarly, wishful thinking has no place in diagnosis. While it is desirable to be optimistic over the outcome of therapy, such optimism, in fact, may stir up false hopes in both parents and child and make eventual disappointment all the greater.

Above all, the psychologist should give a differentiated, rather than an oversimplified, picture of the child. When he describes how a child thinks, feels, and acts, he must do more than focus only on the dominant trends. He must be sensitive to the less explicit, more muted aspects which may be different—and perhaps even opposed—to the dominant trends or to the theoretical mold which makes everything fit into place, at least with our present understanding. Thus, it is not enough to report that a child has hostile, destructive, and hateful feelings toward adults if, at the same time, there is evidence that he also has admiring, respectful, and affectionate ones.

The psychologist, of course, cannot report everything that he sees—some kind of order and limit must be imposed on the mass of data. But he does a disservice both to the child and to members of his team when he avoids the complexity of his observations. Frequently, finding the optimal point between what should be included and what should be left out is one of the most difficult problems the psychologist must resolve in writing his report.

A final suggestion: It is usually unwise to share specific test findings with parents, particularly in cases of mental retardation. Often when a psychologist comes to the parents with a report of their child's specific behavior on tests that he was unable to pass, the parents respond by saying that their child can do very similar things at home. What they do not understand, of course, is that the circumstances under which a child is tested are very special, including the fact that the tests are given in a different environment from the home and are constructed according to very careful specifications. In desperation, the parents often need to deny the validity and significance of the tests and seize hold of any opportunity to do so. For this reason, the psychologist usually avoids this kind of problem by stating the child is unable to do those things that other children his age are able to do.

Of course, the issues involved in the diagnostic testing of

children will include far more than our brief discussion can possibly indicate. However, our aim has been to present a point of view rather than a manual. Hopefully, the reader will find this point of view helpful in approaching the almost always complex task of testing children as part of the diagnostic process.

CHAPTER V

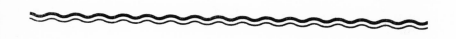

Speech, Language, and Hearing

Speech, language, and hearing together constitute a means of communication unique to human beings. Understanding the variations possible in speech, language, and hearing enhances and deepens our understanding of an individual. While these elements of communication represent only part of any person's emotional, intellectual, and social behavior, they involve some of the most important skills anyone possesses.

The clarification of how speech, language, and hearing both affect and reflect the individual's total adjustment is the unique contribution offered to the psychiatric team by the speech pathologist.

Before we present specific examples of this unique contribution, a brief consideration of the speech pathologist's basic assumptions may be helpful, especially since the usual members of a psychiatric team are not too familiar with his work. This lack of familiarity is due not only to the confusion of many professions about his working assumptions but also because of lack of experience with using the kind of data he gathers in a total psychiatric evaluation.

The speech pathologist assumes that speech, language, and hearing not only are affected by but reflect an individual's environment (especially his interaction in his family), his organic endowment, and his psychological functioning. As a result, he considers communication behavior to be a complex which can never be entirely reduced to just phonetic, or just physiological, or just neurological, or just psychological factors alone. Evaluations of speech, language, and hearing may emphasize some of these factors as being of prime importance in individual patients, but they can never exclude the fact that all factors must be present and have some balance if normal verbal communication is to occur.

The guidelines used in labeling communication as deviant can best be introduced by a definition of speech, language, and hearing disorders. But, first, let us stress that the label *defective speech* is never used for colloquialisms or regional dialects. Likewise, the normal developmental errors made by children during their first seven to eight years of life are never considered speech defects, though they may possibly reflect the child's reactions to transitory environmental stress. Excluding these variations, we can say that speech does become defective when, as a result of the way a person articulates his sounds, he cannot adequately and smoothly convey his thoughts to his own or others' satisfaction. Language is considered disturbed when the child fails to use sounds to develop words having the symbolic meanings usually ascribed by society or when there is a breakdown in the language of an already normally functioning child as a result of

some form of cerebral insult. A disturbance in hearing occurs whenever there is a significant interference with the ability to monitor
through listening to oneself, to other individuals, or to the sounds
of the environment. Hearing may be impaired either because of
organic or functional reasons, or both.

With these simple concise definitions in mind, we can move
on to show how the major determinants of verbal communication
are reflected in specific cases and how the material gathered by the
speech pathologist can deepen the usual diagnostic picture obtained
of a child.

FUNCTIONS OF INTERACTION

The influence families exert on the function of speech,
language, and hearing is usually underestimated. Within this group
the child hears the majority of his early sounds and responds to
them with his own sounds. The pleasant and unpleasant affect that
becomes associated with these sounds shapes, to a large extent, the
ways in which he eventually receives sounds and expresses himself
through the medium of sound. The following excerpt, given by a
mother of a retarded child who was not yet speaking, illustrates
how negative affect may become associated with the development
of a child's speech and language.

> *Case Example:* Mrs. M. first described her six-year-old
> son J.'s jealousy when she feeds his baby sister or gives
> her attention and his inability to let himself be cuddled
> or held, since he is a wriggly, restless child. Mrs. M. also
> said that when his sister responds to being talked to, J.
> gets angry. He gets angry (according to his mother) be-
> cause he cannot talk and cannot make known his wishes.
> However, she reported that all attempts at getting him to
> talk have been to no avail. Mrs. M. expressed anger and
> the feeling that if he wanted to talk he could, but simply
> refuses to do so.

This account is typical of that which many mothers and fathers
give in discussing their child's delay in acquiring language or

disturbance in speech or hearing. In such homes the sounds of language have become imbued with so many negative feelings that the function of a sound as a medium of communication has been pushed in the background.

Speech, language, and hearing begin to develop early. Many people think speech and language are functions that will not be observed for at least the first year of a child's life. However, both experience and research indicate that it is extremely important how the parent uses sound and encourages the child to use sound during those first twelve months. Providing a child with only physical necessities has a devastating effect on the development of communication even among children who are not retarded and not institutionalized. The effect is easily illustrated.

> *Case Example:* A two-year, nine-month-old girl was referred for a psychiatric evaluation because her parents were concerned over her lack of language development and her overaggressive and destructive tendencies. They also reported that she has her own private language. The only time it becomes readily intelligible is during a drowsy state of being almost but not quite asleep. Speech and language usage within the home consists of yelling and pointing whenever she wants something. Whenever she is not understood, she will shove her plate on the floor or act in some other aggressive way. The speech evaluation disclosed that she did not use either speech sounds or language in interpersonal communication. Both her mother and father largely ignored her during her first year of life. The mother's illness, which consumed most of her waking thoughts and caused her to be separated from the child for a month during this first year, and pressures on the father to complete graduate school served as the ostensible reasons. Complicating interaction with this child from the parent's and relative's view was the fact that during this same first year she was in a cast for a few months to correct a congenital hip defect. The cast became urine soaked, and the mother and father reported

being repelled by the odor. During the time she was in her cast, the mother reported her child made "no demands for attention." The parents have continued to be unable to respond to the girl. The mother feels the child is distant in her relationships, unable to be close to her, and deliberately acts this way to express anger toward her. The parents see her as being difficult to manage and less appealing than their other daughter. This feeling was echoed by others in her environment, such as the grandparents and neighbor children. Clinical examinations by the neurologist and psychologist revealed no evidence of symbolic disturbance, and they felt she functioned at least between the two- and two-and-a-half-year level from an intellectual standpoint. Language, although infrequent in its use, was, when present, similar to that seen in a child between two to three years of age. There was no hearing loss. Although there was a mild impairment of tongue movement, it was not sufficient to explain her poor use of speech.

This case illustrates the effect of a family's disturbed interaction during a crucial period in the development of communication. It is our impression that such descriptions would be more the rule than the exception for families having children normal in all respects except for a slow development of speech and language. In studying the family's effect on speech and language development, such factors as the amount of cooing and babbling and the amount of time spent by the parents in reciprocal communication seem to be important factors. Our experience has led us to believe that a parent who has time to interact verbally during a child's infancy is likely to be a parent who later has time to respond to other forms of communication used by a child, whether verbal or not.

Of course, the thesis which we have developed up to this point is difficult to prove since concern about the welfare of the child would demand some sort of intervention were the case called to your attention. However, it is possible to see a family's communication patterns in daily life and to reconstruct through the family history the conditions which must have been present earlier. One way of validating our inferences is to observe a family interacting together. We can arrange this situation by asking them to talk and do things together in a large room where we can observe them by means of a one-way mirror. The primary purpose of such an observation is to obtain samples of communication while a child is within the family setting. An excerpt from a report on one such observation of a five-year, ten-month-old girl and her parents is illustrative.

> Case Example: One might characterize this girl's speech environment as one in which there is a hailstorm of adult command, countercommand, and negative remarks which abate only from the need of the parents to catch their breath. In this fleeting time the child is supposed to contribute a yes or no but nothing more. Such an environment would almost totally inhibit spontaneous formulation of language, encourage rejection of sound, and make it necessary for her to use the speech and language she has in a defensive manner. Her periods of unintelligibility may be understood as regressions in communication under stress.

This vignette proved to be an accurate representation not only of the child's speech and language behavior but also of parental interaction as confirmed by the caseworker's findings.

Equally important to the child's development of adequate communication is the parents' interpretation of how much he hears. A child incorrectly considered as odd and deaf by parents almost from the moment of birth is likely to have only intermittent psychological reception of language or, at the least, disturbed sensitivity for sound. One set of parents we saw reported almost this very situation. That is, they felt their child from birth to be queer and latched on to the explanation of deafness as a cause. Although the child did have a peculiar congenital hearing loss which caused a true deficiency in the lower frequencies, he also had sufficient hearing to understand at least part of the incoming language. When tested by pure-tone audiometric procedures, he completely refused to respond to any sound except at extremely high intensity. Yet, his teachers reported he frequently responded to oral language of an abstract nature, indicating that he was hearing and comprehending material. He was treated as a deaf child by his parents and relatives and sent away to a school for the deaf early in life. At the time of the diagnostic evaluation, he was fourteen years old. The psychiatric study revealed among other things that when he feels under particular pressure to accomplish something, he negatively and actively shuts a person out. How this form of behavior and the influence of parental rejection influenced him to adopt the role of being profoundly deaf was extremely subtle and hard to clarify during the evaluation. However, the team recommended psychiatric treatment and is still following his case.

FUNCTIONS OF ORGANIC ENDOWMENT

Perhaps because observing and labeling organic factors is relatively easy, they are frequently overemphasized as causes of disturbed communication. A prime example is seen in the number of frenums clipped in hopes that the child's speech will improve; many laymen and professional people think that a tongue capable of all sorts of gyrations is the most significant thing necessary for developing normal speech. Actually, only a minimal amount of movement is necessary. Two organic conditions which do affect speech are impaired coordination of tongue movement and a cleft palate. A description given by a speech pathologist for a child with a significant neuromuscular problem of the tongue is as follows:

> *Case Example:* John, age five, is unable to elevate his tongue adequately for speech. He has poor velo-pharyngeal closure resulting in nasal speech, and the test of diadochokinesis utilizing the various speech articulators shows gross disturbances. In addition, he is sometimes momentarily unable to initiate phonation. His parents report that he has trouble chewing and swallowing foods and will not eat chewy meats of any kind. There seems

to be an almost total lack of movement of the styloglossus muscle. He is not tongue-tied.

The speech produced by such a child is properly labeled *dysarthric speech*. Although the term *dysarthria* is used to describe all speech defects by some professions, speech pathologists generally reserve it to indicate only speech disturbed as the result of some defect in neuromuscular functioning. The child in the case example above lived in a remote farm community where his speech handicap had not yet become too significant in his interaction with other children or with adults. His parents, brothers, and sisters understood him and, since he was the youngest, had adjusted the family routine to him. Valuable time had been lost by his not having been referred for help earlier. By integrating the findings of the speech pathologist with those of the neurologist, it was possible to plan a program for this boy which would hopefully allow speech and language to develop in a relatively satisfactory fashion.

Another physical deviation which affects development of speech is the presence of a cleft palate or cleft lip. Although surgery is often performed early on the lip, much more time, in a relative sense, passes before the palate is usually closed. In the meantime the child needs to experiment in making sounds, and he does so in atypical ways. Of course, such compensatory action depends on the extent of the cleft. At any rate, by the time surgery is completed, the child will already have used many atypical physiological patterns of articulation. Not to be discounted in this entire picture is the reaction of the child's parents and peers. As indicated earlier, parental acceptance of use of speech is extremely important for normal speech development. In such physical disturbances as the cleft palate, parental acceptance of communication attempts by children is even more important. Speech pathologists use many diagnostic techniques in studying the physiological adequacy of children with an organic deviation like the cleft palate. Analysis of sounds dependent upon normal functioning of the velum and pharyngeal wall by X-ray cinematography are helpful in determining the adequacy of a child's physiological mechanism. However, even where a definite physical anomaly exists, there is also a need to consider the meaning to the child of his being able to communicate. This aspect is highlighted by the fact that many children with perfectly repaired anatomical structures have quite defective speech.

In the area of hearing, the importance of normal structures is self-evident. However, some remarks are in order. Speech and language can be understood adequately when only one ear has normal auditory functioning. Measurement of hearing loss is usually done by audiologists. Audiology has evolved into a separate profession because of the special background required in psychophysics, acquaintance with the medical aspects of hearing loss, and knowledge of electronics. However, in our setting, the speech pathologist performs some of the audiologist's basic functions by determining in a gross way if a measurable disturbance in hearing exists. If so, an appropriate referral is made for further testing and study by the otologist and audiologist. Helpful steps in identifying the extent of hearing loss include tests of hearing by pure tones and speech. The stimuli are administered by air conduction and bone conduction to the individual child. In addition to conventional audiometric procedures, audiologists also study electrodermal and electroencephalic responses to sound.

FUNCTIONS OF PSYCHOLOGICAL FACTORS

Many may consider this section the main focus of the chapter. Undue focus on this area is, however, as fallacious as undue focus on the earlier sections, for our thesis is that all of these areas determine the manner of speaking and hearing. As a result, it will be necessary to discuss the relationship of both external and internal psychological factors in communication within a broad framework that will re-emphasize the contribution of the family, the environment, and organic endowment.

A most important dimension of any psychological evaluation is intellectual functioning. The relationship of intelligence to speech and language is illustrated by the following case.

Case Example: A five-year, ten-month-old boy was referred to the Menninger Clinic because of his poor response to past psychotherapy. Part of the task to which the psychiatric team directed its attention was trying to define the relative roles of a severe emotional disturbance of autistic proportions and mental retardation, both of which had been said to be present in the child in diagnostic studies done elsewhere. Psychological examinations conducted by the psychiatrist and psychologist emphasized the likelihood that the boy was basically a severely defective, organically damaged child. However, sufficient doubt remained because of the child's age, so that the psychiatrist and psychologist hesitated to commit themselves to a final diagnosis.

Observation of his speech sounds suggested that he used sounds with no greater facility than that of a child one year old or younger. At this level his sounds were used to promote relationships and to establish contact with people in his environment. He also gave clear evidence of responding to sound in the primitive fashion expected of a child around one to one and a half years of age. His voice quality was not suggestive of a deaf child, nor did any evidence indicate significant neuromuscular involvement of the speech articulators. These findings supported the psychiatrist's and psychologist's finding of severe mental deficiency as the basic disturbance.

A relationship between intellectual functioning and articulation skill may also be present in a child who is not so severely retarded. Articulation skills are studied by means of standardized tests. Here at the clinic, the Templin-Darley Test of Articulation is used. In this test, the child either names a picture or repeats after the examiner a word which the picture normally evokes. The word contains the sound to be tested. Specifying the age level of articulation ability often adds additional information and confirmation to the psychologist's impression of a child's intellectual functioning. The case of a six-and-a-half-year-old boy illustrates this point.

Case Example: The psychological examination revealed Bill to be retarded, with an IQ of 54 on Form L of the Revised Stanford-Binet. Neurological study showed a mildly abnormal EEG. The neurological diagnosis was "encephalopathy, congenital, cause not clear." Casework revealed a disturbed family, with the father exhibiting paranoid behavior and expressing a great amount of anger toward the child because he was not normal.

Studies of the functioning of his speech mechanism showed it to be adequate for normal speech. There was no hearing loss. The speech evaluation revealed he was articulating sounds at approximately the level of a three-and-a-half-year-old child—a level quite commensurate with his intellectual functioning. In addition, he manifested periods of unintelligible speech, which seemed to be related to external pressures and his reaction to them. This became quite apparent as he was observed in interaction with his parents. That is, his speech became most unintelligible when they directly or indirectly pressured him.

Articulation ability is also modified by maturation. We can illustrate this by a case example.

Case Example: Peggy, age fourteen, had a Full-Scale IQ of 72 as measured by the Wechsler Intelligence Scale for Children. She had been referred because of difficulties in schoolwork, social ineptness, and depression, which had become more acute since entering high school. Although the parents treated their daughter like an infant, they did offer her some support. She had been previously seen at this clinic at age five and a half because she was stuttering. At that time, she was characterized by the examining psychiatrist as unusually fearful and as using compensatory efforts to counterbalance her organic limitations. Shortly after the first consultation, she stopped stuttering. Although the question of why she stopped stuttering is an intriguing one, we will wait until later when we will discuss the possible personality factors affecting stuttering.

The current speech evaluation revealed errors which were not present all of the time. Under stress, she seemed to revert to the use of infantile sounds and a lisp, but generally she was doing well in her speech. No formal speech therapy had been given, and basically she seemed to show good speech intelligibility.

From our experience we can state that given time, relatively few complications, and an IQ of at least 70, the chances are strong that a child will spontaneously correct any difficulties in articulating sounds. With the presentation of this illustration, a qualifying remark should be added. This case was not included to give the impression that a mildly retarded child should have speech therapy deferred until he has had a chance to grow out of the problem. The preceding examples imply that intelligence is one factor which must be considered in trying to understand speech production. Sometimes speech therapy has beneficial effects on retarded children and sometimes it is better to defer it. Even if a child may be likely to grow out of his speech problems, the social and emotional penalties he sustains in the process make intervention for speech therapy in many cases mandatory. Speech therapy with retarded children facilitates their orderly acquisition of speech and helps them cope with problems caused by having poor communication ability.

Let us stress, too, that the results of a speech evaluation do not always agree with reports from other members of the psychiatric team. There is, of course, no inherent reason why the speech pathologist's report must always corroborate other findings, just as there is no certainty that the evaluation by the psychologist, psychiatrist, or neurologist will necessarily support the others' reports. Instead, whether the observations are the speech pathologist's or those of other team members, each new observation is considered one more clue which the group can use to further understanding of a child.

Case Example: A seven-year-old boy who was brought to the clinic for an evaluation because of the increasing demands he made and because of the emptiness and vagueness in his relationships was felt by the psychiatrist and the psychologist to be severely intellectually deficient (IQ estimated at about 40) and to be exhibiting a variety of psychotic-like adjustment patterns. Although the speech examination disclosed many substitutions of a wrong sound for the correct one, his overall articulation pattern was that of a boy of average intelligence. This was obviously in disagreement with the psychological tests and observations reported by the other team members. Of course, the child's level of functioning was undeniably depressed and any treatment plans would have to take this into consideration. Further, the possibility certainly exists that some factor operating in this child allowed a retention of skill in one area even though all other areas were depressed.

By now it is apparent that we believe more than the level of intellectual functioning is expressed in the speech of children; in addition, we also believe that a speech analysis reflects a child's emotions. This possibility should not be surprising since verbal language and expressive sounds are not only a means for individuals to relate to their environment but also the primary way for them to express their needs and feelings. If we regard slips of the tongue as psychologically significant and determined, it is not too large a step to view substitutions of one sound for another as an extension of the same behavior. The problem then becomes how to translate this view into a method for making meaningful observations for use in understanding the child (Rousey and Moriarty, 1965). In the absence of significant neurological findings or neuromuscular involvement of the speech articulators, the inconsistent substitution of one sound for another sometimes appears to us to have psychological meaning. Examples of these may encourage others to consider this point of view. The presence of a lisp (a substitution of the sound *th,* as in *thank,* for the *s* in *sit* or *city*) appears to occur more often in adult females than males and often in individuals who want to remain immature. Demonstrations also indicate that a whistle accompanying the production of this *s* sound frequently occurs when a person is under stress. At the present time, certain sounds appear more productive to observe than others. For example, the manner in which the *s,* the *th,* the *r,* and the *l* are articulated are the most productive sounds for a diognostician to observe.

Study of how a child makes sounds and the particular sounds he makes is also being carried out with seriously disturbed children who cannot cooperate for formal speech evaluations but who do speak in a spontaneous manner. For example, a description of a child's use of sound may allow the speech pathologist to arrive at an estimate of any regression or lack of development in his use of speech. Normative data are available on the use of vowels and consonants through the thirtieth month of life, as well as from age three to age eight. By the thirtieth month of life, the relative percentage of use of the various sounds in the English language approaches that of the adult. By obtaining an adequate sample of the sounds used, it is possible to plot a profile of a child's level of use of sounds.

Another dimension of speech which in our clinical experience seems to reflect the general personality of an individual is voice quality. Wide variations of voice quality are accepted by our society. In fact, these variations are so wide that those observed in a child are often overlooked by clinicians when they might serve as subtle indicators of a child's emotions and feelings. Perhaps part of the reason for this omission is that standardized terminology is not available, and, as a result, the usual recourse is to invoke the nomenclature of the singing profession—a nomenclature not universally negotiable even among educated persons. However, there are some basic categories of voice which appear useful to observe in any evaluation. For example, the child with an unusually high or unusually low pitch is not difficult to label. The phenomenon of high pitch sustained beyond pubescence and in the absence of organic deviations seems to occur usually among boys whose masculine identification is shaky. Even here exceptions exist, and the presence of organic pathology always needs to be considered. Referral to a laryngologist is sometimes indicated. A striking symptom which we have observed rather commonly in psychiatric patients is a hoarse voice. Persistence of a hoarse voice over a long period of time may, for example, indicate some organic pathology, such as vocal nodules or carcinoma of the larynx. It may also have psychological implications, as the following illustrates:

> *Case Example:* The patient, a fourteen-year-old boy, was referred because of increasing behavior disorders. The most pronounced feature about his communication abilities was a definite hoarse voice. This difficulty had persisted since age five. He had had no periods in which he had lost his voice entirely and he had had no special help for this condition. For the purpose of studying some of the possible dynamics in the problem, he was asked to put on a puppet show with a mother, father, boy, and girl puppet. When talking as a father doll, his voice continued to show hoarseness. When talking as the boy doll, his voice dramatically improved and no hoarseness was present. During the observation he also played a game of war with toy soldiers which were present. As the mock battle grew more severe, there was also a noticeable lessening of hoarseness, suggesting that it might also be expressive of the feelings he was discharging during this play. With regard to the continued hoarseness exhibited while playing the part of the father, the psychological examination supported the thesis that he was in the midst of continuing oedipal struggles which he had never resolved.

Another sample of conflict as shown in the voice occurred in a twelve-year-old girl who had been referred because of increasing behavior problems in school and loose thought processes. One of her overt acknowledgments was that she would rather be a boy. Analysis of her voice quality strongly suggested the fact that she indeed was expressing this wish in her voice, for she spoke at such a low pitch that her voice sounded hoarse and rough. The pitch range of her voice was less than half that seen in the usual child of her age. While this part of the speech evaluation high-lighted this aspect of her conflicts, her behavior observed in the examination by other team members helped us to understand her from other viewpoints. (Of course, this is the point we would emphasize over and over: speech, language, and hearing are only parts of a total evaluation and have merit because they deepen findings of other members of the diagnostic team and suggest other areas of importance.) Other forms of voice variation useful to describe and relate to psychological dimensions are nasality, the sound made by talking through the nose, and denasality, the sound made by a person with nasal congestion.

Saved for the last in the discussion of how psychological factors may affect speech is the behavior referred to as stuttering, which in the following discussion is considered synonymous with stammering. As a rule, too many professional people continue to look for a single factor as a cause of stuttering and are unaware that it may be not only a symptom of complex underlying emotional con-flicts but also evidence of bona fide neurological difficulty. This communication difficulty often varies not only from patient to patient but is also variable in the same patient from time to time. The speech pathologist studies and describes the exact nature of such difficulties with the hope that this description can give leads to possible underlying etiological factors, thus making a more rational and comprehensive therapeutic intervention possible.

In individuals who are stuttering severely, verbal and physi-cal behavior takes many strange forms. One twelve-year-old boy felt that every time he talked he had to be careful of "the thing." "The thing," which was his name for stuttering, caused him to make sounds he didn't mean and to employ movements and rituals that he believed would enable him not to stutter. One of the types of rituals employed by stutterers is illustrated in the following:

> *Case Example:* When given a Rorschach card, the patient (mentioned above) made clucking, grunting, and whin-ing noises; next, he put his head on his arms; and, finally,

he pecked with an eraser at the Rorschach card. There were some variations during the testing in his response to materials. These included turning his head away from the examiner, raising his eyebrows, talking in a monotone, raising the pitch of his voice in the middle of a word, and shaking his feet rapidly. Psychological testing of this boy suggested he manifested a borderline thought disorder of early adolescence with paranoid trends.

For some children who stutter, and for some of their parents, unconscious needs seem to be fulfilled by this deviant behavior. These processes, however, may often interfere with beginning or sustaining treatment. The following case report illustrates some of the problems which arise both in evaluating a child who stutters and in working with his parents. The excerpt is from a speech pathologist's report of an interview with a twelve-year-old who stuttered and a separate interview with his mother. The consultation ended in a referral for a full psychiatric study.

Case Example: Although this child is a pronounced stutterer, his motivation for receiving help for his problem and his family's motivation for following through is questionable. For example, when I asked him to tell me the things which most troubled him, he replied, "Just my brother, then this danged cold, and then my speech difficulty." The mother felt so ambivalent about getting help she at one point implied that if I continued asking questions, she wouldn't come back. She amplified this communication further by saying, "It's costing me too much now to get help for my boy." Her actual outlay of cash at that point was fifteen dollars.

The same general interaction continued throughout the full-scale psychiatric examination, and the process was eventually terminated by the parents even though they were told special reduced rates for therapy would be available in keeping with their financial means.

Sometimes, a child is referred with the description that he

does stutter. Then it is often hard for various examiners to say he does not. For some reason, use of the label condemns the normal hesitations occurring in everyone's speech to acquire the label of stuttering. The report written by the speech pathologist on one ten-year-old boy illustrates this point: "It is doubtful he would have been labeled a stutterer by any of the diagnostic team if he had not been previously so labeled. His speech patterns are similar to those used by any normal speaker who is temporarily disrupted. No covert or overt behavior usually seen in stuttering was present."

As a result of the speech examination, the rest of the examining team focused their attention in other areas. This allowed a sharp focus on his emotional problems uncontaminated by the attempt to integrate his so-called stuttering into his total behavior pattern.

The effect of psychological factors on a child's use of language is difficult to evaluate. Investigators have just begun to assess this aspect. In addition, problems of terminology cloud the issue when the patient is a child. For example, some professional people hesitate to use the term *aphasia* in describing a congenital lack of language development in a child. We hold that the usefulness of the term with children outweighs any semantic issues. However, the problem of assessing how psychological factors interact with an assumed congenital aphasia is so difficult as to make discussion almost impossible. The diagnosis of childhood aphasia necessitates a careful sorting out of other factors like hearing loss, serious psychological states such as autism, and mental retardation. However, full discussion of the differential diagnostic process in diagnosing childhood aphasia would necessitate a book-length treatise and not just a few paragraphs.

It is, of course, highly unlikely that a child would be aphasic only. Though he need not have other disabilities, he might possibly be retarded or he might have serious emotional difficulties. Our description of one six-year-old child thought to have some receptive and expressive language difficulties illustrates some of the problems.

Case Example: His use of expresive language was spotty

and inconsistent. The only expression he used with any consistency was "more." This was used in conjunction with a game involving physical contact such as tickling and being picked up and held. However, his parents report a series of expressions which he uses and some single words which occur in a spontaneous but often inconsistent and unexpected way. These include such expressions as "don't cut," "don't touch," "don't break it," "no-no," "balloon," "hello," "light bulb," "baby cry," "broke it," and "I'll bite." More complicated attempts at speech on his part result in a jargon. On different occasions this examiner heard him attempt what seemed to him four- to five-word sentences. Although these efforts were unintelligible, he felt they actually occurred; this opinion was based on the intonation patterns and phrasing of the child's jargon. His most typical attempts at communication involve screaming whenever he is frustrated or wants something. For example, his parents report that he screams when he drives by a store where he knows there are balloons and that he screams when he sees candy and wants some. Possibly, over the years, he has reduced the amount of verbal output that he would ordinarily give because he does not receive any reward for doing it. During my second appointment with him, he was decidedly echolalic and would repeat the last word or two of simple expressions used in communicating with him. He did this when talking about a toy gun which he had broken.

In the past, some question arose as to whether or not he was deaf; not infrequently, this is the complaint about children whose comprehension of symbolic language is in some way disturbed. The possibility of deafness, however, had been evaluated and ruled out by audiologists at a university medical center. There was normal voice quality present, which also suggested no major hearing loss.

He understands commands and remarks in a con-

sistent manner. He was able to respond to simple pro-
hibitions during our playtime and would respond to a
single request on the part of his parents during our observation of them. However, there was an unusual amount
of delay between his hearing the request and his responding to it. At home the parents report that he understands
such sentences as: "Sit down," "Go in and eat," "Hang
up your coat," "Pick it up and put it on the table,"
"Get in your room," "Go to the backyard," "Stay out
of the street," "Close the windows," "Plug in the sweeper
cord," "Turn off the switch," "Put on your shoes [also
other items of clothing]," and "Put the silverware on the
table." Although he comprehends more when gestures
are used, he in turn does not use gestures as effectively
as he might to communicate his thoughts.

He responded well to having only one to two toys
in the room. He was not destructive and aggressive
toward me during these times. It would seem that both
the type and amount of physical and verbal stimuli are
important factors in controlling his hyperactivity and resulting destructiveness. During my times with him, he
was most at ease and pleasant when we related in a
physical sense. That is, he enjoyed my picking him up,
setting him on my lap, and tickling him. He repeatedly
asked for "more" and retained this concept over the
period of our appointments. However, despite this level of
communication, there was a certain detachment in our
relationship.

The psychological examination suggested he had
an immature ego which prevented him from controlling
primitive id impulses and maintaining a feeling of self-
identity and stability in the world outside himself. His
intellectual functioning varied from a two-year to a six-
year level. Further complicating a full understanding of
the child was an extremely disturbed family in which both
parents were immature, the father an alcoholic and the

mother dominant and aggressive but also tending to feel rejected and unloved.

Utilizing the observations of the speech pathologist, the examining team helped the family get their boy started in a rehabilitation center where the language disability could be explored further and the parents could receive help for themselves.

A final area which can be affected by psychological factors is the area of hearing. Clinically, most psychiatric personnel would readily agree that the typical psychiatric patient does not use his hearing effectively. Although normal auditory sensitivity as measured by pure-tone audiometry may be present, the ability to hear and understand speech is often disturbed. The necessity for measuring the amount of loss becomes crucial since a mild loss of the ability to understand language can create marked difficulties in educational progress as well as in development of relationships. As mentioned earlier, special equipment is needed for an adequate evaluation of this aspect. However, certain screening procedures can be done which will allow referral to audiologists and otologists where necessary. In one consecutive series of thirty children who were seen for outpatient psychiatric study—regardless of whether there were complaints of hearing difficulties or not—fifteen were found to have difficulty in differentiating sameness and difference in incoming sound stimuli. One child had a probable conductive hearing loss, which was referred to an otologist; another had a fluctuating pattern of hearing loss, which presumably was related to psychogenic factors; and still another had abnormal tone decay, which was absent upon retest at an audiological center after three months of psychotherapy. A complete exploration of hearing abilities in a psychiatric population has never been undertaken. This represents one of the real challenges which must be met in the future.

Of importance in any chapter of this kind is a discussion of the rationale used for deciding whether a child with speech difficulties and emotional problems should have speech therapy and, if so, whether he should have speech therapy along with psychotherapy. An initial consideration is whether the speech or hearing difficulty is *always* present. If it is not, the chances of its being resolved during the process of psychotherapy would appear greater than when the contrary is the case. If the speech difficulty is always present, speech therapy concomitant with psychotherapy may be indicated.

A related issue which forms the nucleus of our second consideration is whether the speech handicap can be related to either internal or external areas of conflict. If so, the decision would usually be to defer speech therapy until progress has been made in psychotherapy. Also implicit in this second consideration is whether or not the speech difficulty has assumed a degree of autonomy independent of any psychiatric problem. Another consideration often of clinical importance for progress in psychotherapy is whether the speech handicap will significantly interfere with verbal communication. For instance, a severe stutterer unable to speak except after a minute or two of struggle could profit by some help with communication, along with and in some cases prior to psychotherapy.

Finally, it is necessary to decide whether a continuation of the speech difficulty might prove harmful to the child's speech mechanism. An excellent example of this eventuality is found in the child with vocal nodules. Although they are often surgically removed, voice therapy may also help this condition. Continued misuse of the voice and subsequent growth and regrowth of nodules with continued surgery might eventually damage the larynx to such an extent that normal phonation would be significantly impaired. Hence, a careful decision must be made whether or not to begin speech therapy.

In conclusion, this chapter has focused on the progress of evaluation of the speech, language, and hearing of children. Thus, we have tried to show the type of information which becomes available by considering these aspects of human behavior and how it both supplements and enlarges the perspective provided by the usual psychiatric evaluation of a child. Because of the unique function of verbal communication in any evaluation and treatment, an understanding of the elements of verbal communication becomes important. Disturbances in speech, language, and hearing can seriously affect a patient's emotional, intellectual, and social behavior. In turn, disturbances in the latter functions can also be reflected through speech, language, and hearing.

CHAPTER VI

The Neurological Examination

For many years the Department of Neurology and Neurosurgery at The Menninger Foundation has not only provided neurological consultation but has functioned in a somewhat expanded role as a full member of the team involved in the psychiatric examination of children. This role implies not only cooperation but our increasing understanding of the complexity and variety of problems encountered at the clinic. The purpose of this chapter is to describe some aspects of the neurologist's function in participating in the studies of the Children's Division. Our focus is on the program of examination, other aspects of which form the major portion of this book. Although the neurological examination is performed in this particular setting and under these particular circumstances, it does not usually differ in principle from the neurological examination given elsewhere.

Repeated surveys of our material have demonstrated that approximately 50 per cent of the patients examined in the Children's Division showed evidence of disturbed functioning of the nervous system. Representative data from one of these surveys are presented in Table 2, illustrating the scope of the problems with which the Children's Division is challenged. This pattern varies from year to year, and observations have been made of other uncommon neurological and general medical conditions.

INTERVIEW WITH PARENTS

Obtaining an adequate genetic, environmental, and medical history is requisite to any complete neurological examination. For this purpose, without exception, the neurologist interviews one or both parents of the child under study. As discussed earlier, the parents are also undergoing interviews with a social worker, who later includes a review of the family's medical history in his report. However, this in no way substitutes for the neurological interview; rather, one complements the other in a helpful manner. The data from the parents are scrutinized in relation to all the data from previous and current neurological examinations.

Prior to the examination the neurologist has received from the coordinator of the total evaluation all available advance information, which may include samples and reports of previous electroencephalograms, X-rays, medical data, and psychological and psychiatric data. This information is supplemented by any pertinent new information which comes up in the course of the evaluation. Knowledge of preceding diagnoses obviously serves to enhance the current neurological examination; reports of the previous examinations often raise questions which widen the opportunities for gaining further information from the current study. Laboratory data, such

TABLE 2

Number

1. Encephalopathy, diffuse, congenital (usually with mental retardation)   32

2. Encephalopathy, diffuse, congenital, with convulsive disorder   2

3. Learning disabilities, organic[a]   8

4. Developmental speech disorder   1

5. Chronic chorea, acquired, cause unknown, mild   1

6. Migraine   1

7. Cyclic vomiting (migrainous family background)   1

8. Cerebromacular degeneration, juvenile type   1

9. Diffuse encephalopathy, chronic, progressive, severe, cause unknown   1

10. Diffuse encephalopathy, acquired, chronic, cause unknown   1

11. Convulsive disorder $\frac{1}{50}$

12. Psychiatric diagnosis only   50

13. Still undiagnosed   1

Total   101

[a] This category of diagnosis includes the syndrome of disability in the learning of reading, writing, arithmetic, and variations thereof. These cases are differentiated, as meticulously as possible, from the equally important and well-recognized instances of learning disabilities which are secondary to emotional disturbance.

as X-rays and electroencephalograms, can be critically evaluated and compared with the new laboratory studies carried out at The Menninger Foundation. Since the child is now older, developmental changes or changes in pathology can be assessed.

Quite as important as the above is the preparation of the parents and the child by the team for the neurological examination. The social worker has already discussed this in some detail with the parents, so that they understand just what kind of a physician a neurologist is and just what the details of the procedure are. The child has been prepared by the psychiatrist, with an explanation of what a neurological examination is like, and a description of the laboratory studies to be done. Although the child, as a result, may feel some initial anxiety, it is our experience that with the help of the team he can handle these fears. They are not comparable with the fears that may arise in a child who faces an experience he knows only by name, such as "a neurological examination" or "laboratory tests." In our opinion this preparation of the patient, along with that of the parents, has been a significant factor in helping us achieve a higher percentage of satisfactorily completed examinations than might otherwise be expected.

The interview with the parents, as already mentioned, is usually conducted with both parents, in the absence of the child if he has any degree of comprehension. The child should not hear a detailed discussion of pregnancy, delivery, and other early factors —some of which might be quite abnormal. Occasionally, one of the parents must remain in the waiting room with the child, and in these cases the mother is usually preferred for the interview since she will recall more clearly many of the details of early development. The presence of both parents, however, provides another opportunity and another setting in which to observe the interaction between mother and father and to gain the benefits of their combined memories.

Questioning is brief and concise and is modified according to the individual circumstances of the case. Nevertheless, we feel that close investigation of family background, genetically and socially, with a detailed review of maternal health prior to and during pregnancy, delivery, infancy, and the child's further development, educational history, immunization history, medical history, as well as the review of more specific neurological symptoms are all essential. The neurological interview also serves to let the parents participate in the medical examination of their child; thus they gain confidence from the fact that a comprehensive investigation is being conducted.

The examination of the patient is conducted without the parents' presence whenever possible. This procedure is not inflexible; should the patient develop marked anxiety, one of the parents is promptly brought in to the examining room to help. The great majority of our patients are over the age of five years. For the occasional very young child, under the age of four or five, and for some of the severely handicapped children with brain damage, the presence of one or both parents is quite desirable. These last two categories of children are usually more comfortable in the presence of the parents, their immediate needs can be met more skillfully, and the examination is more productive. All female patients are examined in the presence of a female assistant.

The manner in which the child is gradually introduced to the direct examination situation has also proved to be helpful. He has not only been prepared in advance but has had the experience of seeing one or both parents go, in advance, to talk with the doctor. We feel that this has a beneficial effect, since the sick child sees the type of effort being made to understand him and his problems. Flexibility is observed in performing the examination, but the most commonly used sequence will serve as a model.

After completion of the interview with one or both parents, the child is invited to accompany the neurologist to his office; in most cases he leaves his parents without difficulty. Since reaching the office involves climbing a flight of stairs, the neurologist has the opportunity to observe the child's motor performance, which often provides further clues when brain damage is present. In the office the child is offered a comfortable chair, or is permitted to wander about, look out of the window, or to explore—within limits—if he desires. In the meantime, conversation proceeds, and the neurologist studies some of the child's orientation and information levels, as well as his perception of the examination. He is invited to write and to participate in peeping, kicking, throwing, and so on—"games" that are used to determine dominance. Then, he is led into the hall, which is of sufficient length for various gait and balance tests, as well as for demonstrating his running pattern. Only after these procedures is he introduced to the examining room, where he will undress so the remainder of the examination can be completed. The neurologist can never be in a hurry; his manner is often rather leisurely; yet he feels every moment may produce some type of observation or information. He conveys the feeling to the child that the examination is important—perhaps also pleasant and even fun. Progressive lessening of initial anxiety, interest and curiosity about the procedures, laughter, giggling, and evidence of feelings of friendship toward the examiner are quite common responses. However, some children display bizarre verbal patterns, unusual fears, paranoid ideas, and other symptoms of emotional illness. The majority of children handle themselves reasonably well most of the time in the examining room—largely because of the gradual staging of events and earlier preparation for the examination. The same principles are used to prepare the child for the laboratory situation described below, and have contributed to a successful experience there.

The foundation for examining the patient remains the standard neurological procedure, including the general physical examination and specific tests of the cranial nerves and of the motor, sensory, reflex, and mental functions. In addition, the child's speech is carefully observed and he is given a brief battery of questions regarding orientation for time, place, and person. Dominance of eye, hand, and foot is usually tested. Along with being asked to write, he is also requested to give at least brief samplings of his reading, spelling, and mathematical abilities. More specialized tests, such as audiograms, caloric testing, and visual field studies may be given, and more elaborate investigations, such as pneumoencephalography and cerebral angiography, are carried out when necessary.

LABORATORY PROCEDURES

The laboratory is not a place apart but rather an integrated portion of the total examining situation. A direct link is established with the laboratory by having the child and his parents visit there immediately after the examination by the neurologist. They are made welcome and the premises and equipment are demonstrated to them, with explanations of the various procedures. This type of experience is frequently helpful to the patient, since it may explain many things about which he may have unwarranted fantasies. The parents, in turn, begin to understand that the laboratory staff not only is competent and friendly but functions under firm direction and is tactfully able to manage many difficult situations.

Most children can attempt some form of cooperation, but some are still restless, anxious, and frightened. Even for the latter, obtaining a complete blood count, blood tests for syphilis, urinalysis, and X-rays of the chest, skull, and wrists is not too difficult. However, the recording of an electroencephalogram is a problem of a different order, since this procedure requires that the patient lie quietly, with his eyes closed, for an extended period of time. We also attempt to obtain, whenever possible, a sleeping record, as well as using hyperventilation and photic stimulation. Sedative medication is used selectively and judiciously in a minority of cases, but, usually, proper understanding is of greater value. For example, a ten-year-old girl who was severely disturbed by phobias and anxieties expressed her fears to the technician while her X-rays were being made; he responded by providing consistent support and appropriate responses. Anxiety continued while the electrodes were placed for the electroencephalogram, but by the time recording was started, without medication, the child was resting so quietly that she provided a very nice waking record before spontaneously going to sleep.

After a neurological examination and a visit to the laboratory, it is usually not difficult for the neurologist to recognize the child who has either undisputed or suspected organic brain disturbance and is, therefore, simply incapable of any significant cooperation in the waking state. For these cases, arrangements are further modified to suit the needs of the child. Whenever there is a failure to complete laboratory work—and the electroencephalogram is the test most often inadequate—we immediately schedule time for another attempt later in the week. A higher dosage of sedative medication may be used or different techniques may be tried, the clues for which may have emerged from the initial experience. With these approaches the number of failures in the laboratory is negligible.

The general success in completing laboratory tests is largely due to the skills of our laboratory staff, which includes the secretary-receptionist and several technicians. Although they are technically proficient and have good equipment with which to work, it is their understanding and experience in dealing with children and their parents, both disturbed and undisturbed, which make for a successful laboratory evaulation.

Direct communication between the team doctors and the laboratory personnel is another important consideration. When, for example, the examining psychiatrist anticipates possible problems with the child in the laboratory, he telephones the staff or promptly visits the technicians and discusses his recommendations with them. These might include specific prescriptions for sedation and the methods or approaches to be used in handling a child. The procedure suggested by the psychiatrist is usually formulated in collaboration with the neurologist.

Information is also contributed by the laboratory staff. Members report whenever indicated or requested upon a child's behavior and his reactions to different procedures in the laboratory. Such a report may provide supplementary information such as that given in the case of the ten-year-old phobic girl mentioned above.

Laboratory technicians are interested in every aspect of the child's physical and psychological functions, as their concern with the entire schedule of laboratory tests shows. The complete blood count and chest X-ray are done for obvious and general medical reasons. The yield of abnormality from these particular tests, as from most of the others, is small, but this is not a deterrent in a program devoted to searching inquiry in each patient. Unsuspected abnormalities, such as anemia, suspicious lung lesions, and cardiac abnormalities, have been detected from time to time. The urinalysis includes a battery of screening tests for metabolic abnormalities, such as phenylketonuria. From the X-rays of the skull a variety of abnormalities can be detected, including the more subtle asymmetries and malformations associated with congenital disturbances of the nervous system.

The electroencephalogram has proved to be a very definite help in detecting vague or unrecognized paroxysmal disorders. The following illustrates the way other members of the team, including a laboratory technician, assisted in establishing a diagnosis of paroxysmal disturbance in a complicated situation.

Case Example: The patient was a thirteen-year-old girl who was brought by her parents for an examination because of angry outbursts, loneliness, difficulty in making friends, and the presence of symptoms of a dual personality. An older brother, described as bright, at the time of the girl's birth was a college student. The health of the parents was good, and the mother's pregnancy was entirely normal until spontaneous labor occurred at seven months gestation. Delivery was easy, the child weighing three pounds, seven ounces and in satisfactory condition. She was kept in an incubator, routinely, for one month, by which time she weighed five pounds, five ounces and was permitted to go home. Development was quite normal, and the patient had no learning difficulties in school through the seventh grade, the year before the examination. A left internal strabismus was noted at two and one-half years of age, and treatment was instituted. The condition improved, with the eye turning in only under conditions of fatigue. A few months before arrival at the clinic, corrective glasses had been prescribed for mild myopia. Detailed questioning revealed no recognized symptoms of any paroxysmal disturbance. Psychological symptoms had developed at about eleven years of age when the patient began to talk about an imaginary friend; about eight months before the examination, the patient began to assume the role of the friend, thus manifesting a dual personality by playing different roles at different times. Some time after that, evidence indicated a good deal of actual hallucination, and the patient would spend long periods of time in her room talking to at least one other imaginary friend, this time a boy.

General physical and neurological examinations were entirely normal. Psychological testing revealed a shy, sensitive, alert, and well-oriented girl who had fantasied another world and another personality, escaping into these frequently under stress. Her intellectual level measured on the Wechsler-Bellevue Intelligence Scale revealed a verbal quotient of 126, and a performance quotient of 114, with a full-scale quotient of 114.

Laboratory tests were entirely normal except for the electroencephalogram, which revealed an abnormal, non-focal pattern of whole brain bursts of polyspike and four-per-second slow wave activity, more frequent during sleeping than waking, and also repeatedly triggered by photic stimulation at the fifteen- to eighteen-per-second range, single flash.

Additional information came from the laboratory technician who took a blood sample from the patient. The technician described clearly that in the midst of a distinct and logical conversation, while the blood was being drawn, the patient's speech suddenly became garbled and incomprehensible for a period of five seconds; then it became quite normal, and lucid conversation continued. Further information came from the psychologists, who had observed a number of suspicious and extremely brief intervals when the patient seemed to be slightly out of contact. None of these episodes was clear-cut and since they were observed in the midst of many impressive symptoms of psychological illness, no conclusions could be drawn from them alone.

It was also interesting to note that when the patient was escorted to visit the laboratory in the customary fashion after the neurological examination, she stated that she had no intention of taking the tests on the following day, but she did agree to go over and look at the laboratory. After the laboratory tests had been completed, the patient reported to the psychologist that she was able to adapt to the great stress which the laboratory tests caused her by changing to her other personality and permitting her alter ego to undergo the test in place of her real self. Thus, the technician worked with a girl who was relatively calm, cooperative, in good contact, and quite reasonable except for the one brief episode of confusion described above. During the course of further psychiatric examination, a very strong possibility developed that a third personality was involved in the structure of this girl's psychological functioning, indicating multiple, rather than dual, personality.

The final diagnosis included both that of dissociative reaction and of convulsive disorder from an unknown cause. The recommendations included residential treatment and further neurological investigation and treatment of the seizures.

The electroencephalogram can be used as a tool for studying function under a variety of conditions, including those in which drugs have been either withheld or administered. For example, in the next case we shall cite of a nine-year-old girl, electroencephalograms were recorded both while the child was receiving varying doses of certain stimulants and after she had been taken completely off this type of medication. An attitude of search and inquiry from any electroencephalographic techniques which are valid and helpful is maintained.

Under any circumstance, the electroencephalogram recording is subjected to a rigorous interpretation, not only of the tracing itself but of the relationship of the findings to the clinical disorder. The electroencephalogram remains a laboratory test which must be evaluated in terms of the clinical problems. We have a firm feeling that treatment should never be directed to an electroencephalogram tracing but must always be directed, instead, to the patient. However, if an abnormal electroencephalogram is detected in the absence of any clinical correlates (and this occurs in 10 to 15 per cent of the asymptomatic population), it is duly recognized. Adequate follow-up studies of the patient and serial electroencephalography are used, but medication does not advise on the basis of electroencephalographic findings alone.

Routine X-rays of the wrists have been made now for some

time to help detect, through bone-age study, any further indications of disturbance in the growing organism. A variety of other laboratory tests may be used, if indicated, in the individual patient, provided they can be accomplished with relative ease during the examination period. If more extensive tests are still required, the patient is usually referred back to his family doctor. However, the occasional need for more extensive neurological tests, such as pneumoencephalography, may result in an extension of the examination time, with the test performed at the clinic.

> *Case Example:* A nine-year-old girl who had chiefly complained about excessive sleepiness for two years showed normal physical and normal neurological examinations. Electroencephalograms were abnormal, diffusely. The entire situation was extraordinarily complicated by a number of very overt emotional problems. In order to clarify this very complex situation, pneumoencephalography was suggested. This was arranged during the summer vacation period, successfully completed in the usual manner at our local general hospital, and proved to be helpful in ruling out the possibility of any expanding or atrophic intracranial lesions.

Before the total examination time has elapsed, additional specific questions can be asked of parents, additional specific laboratory tests or repeat tests can be given, and special investigations into areas of psychiatric, psychological, or neurological testing can be promptly arranged.

CONCLUSIONS

We have noted that a significant proportion of children brought for a psychiatric examination will have organic neurological disorders. Special "biases" of the neurological examiner can help to diagnose or clarify these conditions—biases which have been reinforced by practical clinical experience.

The complex work of the neurologist requires special concern with the following:

1. Stress upon obtaining a detailed family history of organic disease (complementing the valid emphasis of psychiatrists and social workers on the familial interpersonal relationships).

2. Particular emphasis upon antenatal health of the mother, course of the pregnancy, circumstances of delivery, and descriptions of the first hours and weeks of life.

3. Further attention to stages of acquisition of motor, perceptual, and speech functions.

4. Search for abnormal periodic symptoms, such as alterations of consciousness.

5. Evaluation of possible effects of major or minor head trauma, as well as systemic infections and metabolic disorders.

6. Perception of such pertinent physical findings outside the nervous system as the adenoma sebaceum of tuberous sclerosis, the anomalous auricles and webbed toes of congenital brain malformation and the facies of gargoylism, among numerous others.

7. Performing the neurological examination with ability and experience with children.

In addition to the above concerns, the neurologist can use his experience in synthesizing the entire body of historical, examinational, and laboratory information. He can contribute a challenging role in team discussion of behavioral deviations which may be either organic or psychogenic, or a result of interaction of both organic and psychological factors, such as irritability, fatigability, vomiting, headaches, "spells," drowsiness, and abnormal movements.

Inevitably, a certain number of patients will provide complex problems in differential diagnoses, and the team members' intent is to stress this possibility rather than to underestimate it. They are not reluctant to recognize that classifiable psychiatric disorders may exist in an individual who also shows clearly defined and classifiable neurological disturbances. Overcoming the obstacles which the dichotomy between organic and functional disorders might present in analyzing a clinical problem has often contributed to a clearer understanding of both ranges of disorders. With goals which include a clearer understanding not only of why the child is functioning as he is but how he can be helped with combinations of therapy best suited to his problems, the team seems to function better and to become less involved in nonproductive academic controversies.

In some cases, extended neurological examinations have been requested and completed at varying times after the initial examination, either prior to residential or outpatient treatment or on the occasion of a return visit for re-examination. Repeated neurological examinations have usually been fruitful in respect to clarifying disturbances previously observed, discovering disorders previously unrecognized, or in confirming the status of a previously described condition. The principle of repeated or serial examinations must be maintained and underscores the fact that the neurologist is dealing with a rapidly growing and developing organism. He is faced with the challenge and the responsibility of keeping pace with all phases of development. The concept of extended or continuing examination should, therefore, not be seen as anything unique, but rather as a guiding principle for the neurologist as well as other members of the team.

We feel that the principles involved in neurological examination as we have described it can be adapted to most settings for the psychiatric examination of children. In fact, the child psychiatrist may develop his own neurological talents if a neurological consultant is not available. Social workers or psychologists who may be the first to see the child and his family should develop their abilities to detect clues leading to recommendations for further neurological investigation. In any event, neurological scrutiny is necessary for evaluating a child who is brought for psychiatric examination.

In our experience—as we have stressed earlier—structural disease of or damage to the nervous system is a factor in approximately 50 per cent of patients who are referred to us for psychiatric evaluation. Errors in diagnosis and prognosis, as well as in the recommendations for treatment, will increase if a neurological inquiry is not a part of the total evaluation.

CHAPTER VII

The Psychiatric
Examination

The basic principle guiding the psychiatrist is concisely stated by Erikson (1963) in *Childhood and Society:* "The relevance of a given item in a case history is derived from the relevance of other items to which it contributes relevance and from which, by the very fact of this contribution, it derives additional meaning [p. 41]."

Throughout this chapter, this principle must be kept in

mind; thus the psychiatric examination of a child should be viewed as part of the team process in which material gathered by each member in different segments of the study has relevance to the other data assembled. During the limited period of a week in which the material is collected, insights emerging early in the examination facilitate the emergence of later material as the examination period progresses. The data collected must also be seen in relation to the reactions of the parents who may understate, exaggerate, select, or distort the intrinsic difficulties of their child. Thus, the roles and functions of the examining psychiatrist,* like those of the other examiners, are varied; and they transcend the mere technical procedure of examining the child.

As an examiner, the psychiatrist holds an equal responsibility with each team member—the caseworker, the psychologist, the neurologist, and the speech and hearing pathologist—to integrate the material from all sources, beginning with the initial referral material and ending with the responses of the child and parents in the final postevaluation conference. As a physician, the psychiatrist may sometimes be called upon to use both his medical experience and orientation in the effort to understand all aspects of the evolving picture of the child and his family. His ideas, as well as the data he obtains directly from the child, may also stimulate the other team members to fresh insights, which in turn may wake new understanding of the child and his family. Furthermore, the psychiatrist must be a leader in the final integration of the historical items, the psychological test results, the neurological findings and the results of his own direct study of the child, so as to reach a cohesive, comprehensive, and usable diagnostic picture of the patient. In the process, the psychiatrist needs to be able to conceptualize the interrelationships of the individual with familial,

* This chapter is written entirely in the spirit of the book, that is, the psychiatrist is discussed as a member of a team. Some may wonder to what extent this particular chapter may apply to the psychiatrist functioning in private practice. Some aspects of this discussion of the psychiatric examination of the child may apply to private practice; but since no systematic attempt is made to distinguish which aspects apply and which do not, the reader would be advised to assume the chapter does not apply to private practice.

social, biological, developmental, and maturational factors; thus, he can contribute to the team's assessment not only of the child's present standing in his family but his social setting (culture and subculture) in relation to his current biological, maturational, and developmental stage.

On such an assessment meaningful recommendations may be based. This task, of course, requires that the psychiatrist have the mature capacity and experience to appreciate all team members' contributions, as well as a practical grasp of the force these factors can exert on the total functioning and malfunctioning of the child-patient and his family. Fulfilling this role of leadership requires a step-by-step involvement with the other team members throughout the examination. He cannot hide, as it were, behind the role of seeing the child only, without reference to the family. He must be able to empathize deeply with the child and to recognize his problems, wishes, disappointments, rages, and fears. He may, for example, find it necessary to handle certain material the child has told him in a particularly discreet and confidential fashion. Often he takes a stand in supporting the child's need for professional help. He may make certain technical maneuvers to help the child recognize that he should present his own wishes more clearly to his parents and in this sense free himself from them, relatively. At the same time the psychiatrist must be equally capable of the detachment needed to integrate his findings into the total family picture. Thus he does not allow his concern for the child to interfere with the team process of evaluation.

The goal of the psychiatrist's examination of the child is first of all to develop a valid understanding of the child's psychic structure, style, and functioning. He tries then to gain a picture of the following:

1. The general character structure of the child, while recognizing that in children character is often not yet finally developed.

2. The child's symptoms, if any.

3. The general physical (including neurological) status of the child, checking possible deficiencies in all sensory, motor,

physiological, and neurological zones, the present status and history of his physiological and vegetative functioning, and the possible relation of marked present or past disturbances in these to disturbances of cognitive functioning or aspects of control (to be discussed below).

4. The general maturational level and pattern of the child in terms of balances and imbalances of perceptual and motor skills, general language function, concept development, social interaction, age-appropriate interests, knowledge of the environment, and so on.

5. The general level of the child's drive development, which includes an estimate of the predominant stage of psychosexual development and any particular points of potential, or definite, fixation in the psychosexual development not commensurate with the general level expected at his chronological age. It also includes an estimate of any points of fixation in the development of the aggressive drives of the child not commensurate with the general level of psychosexual development or the chronological age.

6. The general degree of regression of the child, that is, to what extent the regression may be temporary or relatively persistent or recurrent. A virtual arrest of psychosexual development (as seen, for instance, in severely psychotic children) must be distinguished from temporary regression to a lower level of development. It is also necessary to determine as far as possible the degree to which the regression is due to internal and external pressures; the degree to which minimal-to-severe deficit or imbalances of equipment or neurophysiological dysfunction affect the arrest, retardation, or regression; and the relation of the regression to fixation points.

7. The general level of ego development in relation to the level of drive development. This includes a study of the child's ego strengths along with other strengths, and also a consideration of specific ego functions which are overaccelerated or overdeveloped (opposite of regression) in this child. Special areas where ego functioning is particularly defective need to be considered in relation to limitations of resources for compensation and management.

By no means are these goals the only aims of the examination. The child is, after all, a patient, a young human being whom we presume to be suffering emotionally in a current, real life situation. Hence, we may list additional goals as follows:

8. We must carefully assess the current functioning of the child as to the degree of his discomfort and the degree to which such suffering is recognized by the child (ego-alien) as contrasted with not being recognized by the child (ego-syntonic).

9. We also need to describe the details of psychological defense maneuvers employed by the child in his struggle with his discomfort, regardless of whether he is aware of his sufferings.

10. We also need to relate these defensive mechanisms to his psychosexual stage of development and to the general state of his ego functioning (as outlined above). In addition, we need to evaluate the extent to which these defensive maneuvers have brought about what parents have reported as "symptoms" or "complaints."

11. Furthermore, we must observe and describe appropriate samples of his cognitive processes, including such processes as arithmetical computation, time sense, judgment, reasoning, insight, and memory, all of which are important for school adjustment and many everyday tasks.

12. We must evaluate disordered functioning such as distorted ideas or delusional thinking, as well as confusion or extreme fluidity or scatter in thought, in relation to the transitory or chronic stress in which cognitive functioning is disrupted.

13. We need to describe the child's prominent fantasies both as to content, organization, and realism, and as to the reflection in them of defensive maneuvers.

Not only is the child a suffering human being but he is also a young person living with other people who mean a great deal to him and to whom, in turn, he is very important. Hence, in the controlled setting of the psychiatric interview, we may gain the following vital information:

1. The child's modes of relating and the nature of his relationships (object relations) as reflected in apparently typical responses to other people such as the examining psychiatrist, his parents, peers, siblings, and other adults (teachers, authority figures, and strangers, among others).

2. Feelings about himself, including evidence of self-esteem, self-concepts, aspirations for the present and future, ideals, and the relative distance between self-concept and ideals.

3. An estimate as to the balance in the child between a sense of basic trust and of mistrust, between autonomy and shame and doubt, according to the nuclear developmental conflicts described by Erikson (1963).

4. Observations on the child's emotional (affective) responses to other people (including himself)—the nature and degree of anger, of sexual drive, of pregenital impulses such as oral wishes and anal-sadistic fantasies, and of the consequent guilt or depression, or anxiety or fear, or other feelings. In exploring such areas—for example, guilty feelings—we are, of course, considering several aspects of what is usually subsumed under the term *superego*.

The child's reactions to the interview should also provide data on the stress accompanying different points of the discussion and his way of struggling with it. The degree of his acceptance and understanding will also be reflected in his behavior in the interview, as will his feelings about the evaluation process in general (especially as it progresses). The relationship of these emotional reactions to the stage of psychosexual development and ego development, as discussed earlier, can then be considered along with their relationship to the psychological defensive maneuvers used by the child.

Although, in one sense, it is incorrect to separate the category of strengths from the other aspects of the assessment already mentioned, a separate listing has the pragmatic advantage of underscoring one area of the examination so often and so disastrously overlooked. As emphasized frequently in this book, the child who is brought to the clinic for examination is by no means only, or predominantly, a walking textbook of psychopathology. Though perhaps damaged or even deeply disorganized, he nevertheless possesses strengths or assets. He has specific capacities and special ways of coping with his life and himself. These must be recognized during the examination as part of him, of his style, or his endowment. In themselves, they are neither assets nor liabilities; in fact, the same coping methods may have both positive and negative effects on his general adaptation. The coping patterns will vary from child to child and must be related to other aspects of understanding the patient and his parents. This is why we discuss the child's strengths under a separate heading. This list is obviously not to be considered exhaustive. Strengths and assets to be considered include:

1. Ego strength.

2. Personability, including physique, physiognomy, mode of relating to people, and voice quality.

3. General intelligence, especially insight and understanding.

4. The capacity to delay gratification (in which the age and developmental level of the child is to be carefully taken into account).

5. The particular style and resources of the patient in coping with frustration.

6. The capacity to accept substitutes.

7. The capacity for introspection.

8. Special abilities, for example, types of motor skill, artistic talents, musical learnings, and literary abilities.

9. The capacity for sublimation.

10. Determination, persistence, and a capacity to keep struggling.

11. General integrative capacity rather than a disorganization trend; ability to organize his life, to make constructive use of spare time, and to develop positive interests.

12. The capacity to utilize a psychotherapeutic relationship. All the above observations must be organized into an integrated picture of the nature of the child's disturbance, his resources for overcoming it, and his own image of himself as outlined above.

DIFFICULTIES

How does the examining psychiatrist reach the goals we have listed? By what methods does he proceed? Before discussing these questions, we should look at some of the difficulties he faces. First, by virtue of the fact that children grow, he must be prepared for the wide span of their developmental levels. Thus, he must deal with, and relate to, anyone from a toddling two-year-old to a sophisticated seventeen-year-old. But the task is even more difficult since a considerable proportion of children have complex time-tables for growth in different zones of their equipment and functioning. A child who meets all the norms is rare. In addition, the psychiatrist must expect to confront a great variety of patients, ranging from a totally nonspeaking or nonhearing or nonattentive child to a belligerent and terrifying youngster who seems to rush to climb to the top of the nearest and tallest tree (or fire escape); or from a painfully shy, wide-eyed, and charming little girl to an openly seductive or icily furious young woman of sixteen.

Furthermore, although the design of team functioning insulates the psychiatrist from the direct and intense impact of the parents, who may be anxious, thoroughly demoralized, or angry, he may be confronted by them sometime during the week of examination, only to be pushed to the wall with anxious or demanding questions or requests for prolonged reports. During the examination, he must keep a balance between allegiance to the child and duty to the parents, to whom he may represent the whole clinic team. As a father, perhaps, himself, or as an adult, he may empathize with the parents intensely. On the other hand, because he has chosen a career devoted to children, he may feel deeply pulled to do the child justice, perhaps even to "save" him from the "cruel" environment. Such are only brief examples of what his internal and external struggles may be.

THE FIRST INTERVIEW

Before the family arrives, the examining psychiatrist will have read, and assimilated, in a planning conference with the other team members, *all* the material available prior to the current examination. To fail to do so would be neglectful of his professional responsibility.

The planning conference itself should begin to resolve some of the potential conflict among team members, which so often is a reflection of the conflict within the parents themselves or between the parents and child. For example, a team member may feel that some other member is underestimating the child or the stress to

which he may be exposed. The psychiatrist approaches his first
contact with the child with the intention of supplementing and
complementing other material and he expects each aspect of the
team process to facilitate further understanding of different aspects
of the problem.

Since the psychiatrist must approach the child for the first
time with a relatively open mind, his initial review of available
data, regardless of what they indicate, must be as free of prejudice
as possible. He can use the understanding gained from these data,
as well as the planning which proceeded from this material, as a
frame of reference within which to search for the meanings of the
child's communications. In other words, he can use his impressions
as hooks on which to hang certain findings as the interviews progress, provided he does not rely on these impressions so rigidly that
he cannot change and add to them as the examination proceeds.

Naturally, before his first contact, the psychiatrist must free
his mind of other preoccupations. He should be physically rested;
he should have his schedule arranged so as not to feel pressured by
imminent obligations; and he should feel no need to follow any
particular system or to accomplish any particular goal immediately.
In short, he should present to the child a genuine attitude of having
nothing else to do in the whole world but to be with him and to
get to know him.

Techniques

Let us return now to the question of the method by which
the psychiatrist seeks to reach the goals of the examination. As in
all direct psychiatric intervention, this method is an interview
between two people. The person of the psychiatrist himself is the
main tool. However, the psychiatrist often uses an accessory tool
with most children: the play technique. The term *play therapy*
has led to certain misunderstandings to the serious detriment of
both the technique itself and the goal for which it is designed. The
play of the child in the interview and his use of the toys employed
serve as modes of communication. They are not present merely for
fun or even to make the relation with the psychiatrist more pleasant,
at least not as a primary goal. Certain play material, which in-

cludes what we commonly call toys, can provide a very natural and valuable way for a child not only to express himself to the psychiatrist but also to externalize, convey, and even, in some instances, to master certain important problems expressed in fantasies that most children, disturbed and normal alike, share. In general, younger children respond most naturally to the opportunity to use toys. However, play material can even stimulate some adolescents to communicate feelings or problems in a useful way. However, the psychiatrist need not force play material on the child; the toys can simply be available as part of the basic equipment of the examination play-office.

Playroom and Equipment

The so-called examining room will vary according to the clinical setting and the psychiatrist's personal preferences. Unfortunately, in recent years, insufficient attention has been given to planning a well-designed, well-equipped playroom or play-office. We grant that the relationship with the child in the interview is most central to the examination, that a child may be interviewed adequately if necessary even in a regular hospital room. But a properly equipped, properly designed office is a valuable asset for the examination.

Scott (1961) has described one interesting playroom design. Of course, not all child psychiatrists require such a setup. However, allowing for individual preferences, certain standards do exist. The room should be reasonably comfortable for a child. Under the term *comfort* fall such important factors as the size of the room —not so large as to stimulate hyperactivity or so small as to feel confining. The design itself should provide for a room in which the child may not easily hurt himself or the equipment. The response of different children to the same physical setting may be quite helpful to the psychiatrist. He may find it instructive to observe many children's reactions simply to the squares of linoleum or other patterns on the playroom floor.

As to play equipment, a single overriding principle can serve as a guide in its selection: it should lend itself as a medium of expression for the child's thoughts, ideas, and fantasies. Such standard material as pencils, paper, crayons, and scissors meet this criterion. A doll house, not too small to be used easily, and furnished with toy people and furniture, provides the opportunity for the child to play out domestic scenes and important family interactions. Similarly, baby dolls, with accompanying bed, blanket, and bottles allow for the expression of mothering impulses, nursing, feelings toward younger siblings, infantile wishes, and the like. Teddy bears, cuddly animals, and other dolls fulfill some of these needs as well.

Also included should be equipment that allows for the expression of aggressive urges and conflicts around aggression and competition; thus, some type of battle equipment—possibly materials with which a fort can be built and a variety of toy soldiers—should be provided. The child may convey many feelings about competition and aggression, along with concern over submission and defeat, in battles between soldiers, cowboys, and Indians. Conflicts over aggressive impulses and their control are sometimes externalized through play battles between good guys and bad guys. Rubber knives (rubber is preferable to plastic), toy guns that may or may not look realistic, and such mobile equipment as trucks, airplanes, and automobiles are desirable. Standard competitive games—especially those designed for two players only, such as checkers and some card games—may be quite helpful when used to observe competitive behavior. One of the best games is a set of rubber-tipped darts with a dart gun and target. Made from good plastic material, a large punching bag figure that is designed to return to a standing position after being hit is often useful for evoking aggressive feelings toward authorities or peers.

A range of opinion exists as to the type of dolls that should be on hand in the office. Some child psychiatrists may prefer the figures to be as nondescript as possible, allowing the child to project his own character into them. Others may prefer take-apart dolls which have removable genitals and breasts; these may be used with certain special cases. A set of small plastic dolls which represent the usual members of the family and are both moderately indestructible and flexible enough to allow for different postures seems to be satisfactory for playing out family interactions.

Since the play equipment does not exist primarily for the child's entertainment, intriguing and intricate toys have no place in the playroom office; neither do most so-called educational toys. They do not lend themselves to the expression of the child's thoughts and ideas to the degree permitted by the play material just described. The use of complex constructive toys, such as kits for model airplanes or model-car building, probably has little value for examinational purposes. However, the use of quick building materials, such as Lincoln logs, can show muscle coordination, persistence, and frustration tolerance, as well as the child's preoccupation with enclosures, barriers, and shelter.

Materials for younger children should also be included in the play equipment. In the experience of some psychiatrists studying young psychotic or autistic children, the presence of a push toy has had an interesting diagnostic value. Characteristically, these children do not use the toys for the purpose they were designed; rather, they hold the toy, spin it, and become fascinated with the spinning itself. Building blocks of the type often used in nursery schools are not only conducive to the play of quite young children but they may be effectively used by some older children in setting up houses, forts, roads, bridges, and perhaps even barricades or protective fences. Specially designed, large building blocks of lightweight cardboard a few feet square can be valuable for children in constructing big forts.

The psychiatrist should, of course, consider the placement of the objects within the room. There is often a tendency to include too many objects in the playroom. A play-office definitely should include a cupboard where much of the play equipment can remain out of sight from the child, while the toys can easily be brought into the interview as need arises. Some basic equipment may be in sight on open shelves to allow the child to use when he chooses. For examinational purposes his choices can be quite instructive. Toys which usually should not be placed within the child's sight include such materials as finger paints. Although these are useful, they tend to be overstimulating to some children. When indicated, they can be produced.

A sandbox naturally allows younger children to play out

quite a variety of fantasy themes. Some psychiatrists prefer it to be placed away from the main part of the office—in an alcove, for example—in order to allow a degree of selectivity in its use.

In fact, whether the play area should be contained in an entirely separate room or should be in the alcove of a more traditional office is a moot question. If the playroom is not separate, the all-purpose office-playroom certainly should include a standard desk and chairs for the older child-patient, particularly the adolescent. Since patients of various ages may use some play materials at times, these should be available to everyone. In the combined office-playroom, the psychiatrist should certainly have provisions for removing important papers or treasured and breakable objects from the sight and reach of the younger or more destructive child. Dictating machines, perhaps even telephones, may need protection. To be sure, the psychiatrist has the obligation to set limits, but he may present needless temptations by including unnecessary objects in the room. File cabinets, if included at all, should certainly be locked.

One final recommendation: Though the office may not be used exclusively by the particular examining psychiatrist, it should be one with which he is reasonably familiar. He should prepare ahead of time for each child and be responsible for straightening the office following all interviews.

INITIAL INTERVIEW

Whether the examining psychiatrist introduces himself to the parents or is introduced by another member of the clinic is of less importance than the fact that he meets the parents with the child for the first interview. Such a meeting serves several functions simultaneously. The meeting gives an official stamp to the fact that the child is part of the family and that he has been brought by his parents, no matter how resentful he may feel. This particular meeting says, in effect, to the parents and the child that the psychiatrist is interested in the parents as well as the child; however, it also implies that the psychiatrist relates to the child in private interviews as a separate individual. The greeting gives the psychiatrist an opportunity—though he may use discretion as to the timing and the tact of the wording—to acknowledge his general interest in, and even his availability to, the parents during the week of the evaluation.

The most valuable reason for meeting the parents with the child lies in the opportunity for a brief, significant glimpse of their relationships at this important moment of their lives. Probably no other part of the total evaluative process requires more of the psychiatrist's skill or draws more upon his observing capacities than these initial few moments. He must avoid the pitfall of implying that the only thing that matters to him is the child and that, therefore, the parents are unimportant. On the other hand, he must avoid the equally serious danger of having the child recognize him *only* as the parents' agent who has the same attitudes toward him as his parents have. In practice, we recommend that the psychiatrist speak to the parents first—out of the respect they deserve—but in such a way as to include the child in his total recognition of the situation. He may accomplish this by looking at the child momentarily as he begins to greet the parents. Or he may find it helpful to speak to the parents briefly, then to the child, before returning his attention to the parents again. As we have said, this meeting not only requires skill but can also be rich in information about all the members of the family. What is the glimpse of interaction between mother, father, and child just before they realize the examiner has entered the waiting room? Does the child actively compete with his parents for the examiner's attention? Does he momentarily anticipate attention and then withdraw in defeat? Which of the parents is the more forward? How attentive is the child while the examiner is talking briefly with the parents? Do both parents talk? Do the parents signal in verbal and nonverbal ways that they expect the child to misbehave, or to have difficulty in leaving them, or to refuse to talk to the examiner after they leave? Does the mother shake hands? The psychiatrist must be prepared to scrutinize these and many other signs of interaction at the same time as he tries to make all three participants feel important, at the same time as he allays undue anxiety, and at the same time as he reasonably represents the clinic toward which the parents have innumerable, ready-made reactions and about which the child is so deeply curious.

After this introduction, the psychiatrist should in various ways indicate his interest in each member of the family and their part in the examination. He might make some brief reference to what will occur in the next few days of the evaluation. He might explain that he will be seeing the child alone while the social worker is seeing the parents separately. He might mention that he will meet again with the parents in the final joint conference. This discussion generally need not be long, and it should be omitted altogether when the child is especially anxious. Often, if a serious separation problem for the child is anticipated, taking him away too quickly will intensify the anxiety of everyone involved; in the same situation a prolonged discussion can likewise intensify the anticipated separation anxiety. In any event, the psychiatrist should avoid seeming brusque with the parents, on the one hand, and seeming uninterested in the child, on the other, as he and the patient leave the room.

Many clinics allow one of the parents to accompany the child with the examiner to the playroom if undue separation anxiety is obvious or—in most cases—if the child is less than three years of age. This is certainly a humane approach. However, an alternative approach may offer little or no trauma and yet yield even more information, especially in the case of younger children. In this instance the psychiatrist, while recognizing the anxiety of both mother and child, suggests that the child go with him alone. Such a moment provides a genuine opportunity for true teamwork between social worker and psychiatrist. The social worker, while noting the parents' apprehension, stands ready to pick up clues of their readiness to move away from their child. The psychiatrist's function is to act firmly but gently while taking the initiative and leaving with the child. In our experience this team effort, in the long run, relieves anxiety more than the plan of allowing the mother to accompany her child. The psychiatrist may also reassure the parents that if the child soon becomes too distressed, he can be returned or they can be brought to his office.

In those instances in which the mother has to come with the child, the psychiatrist can suggest that she gradually and quietly leave the patient after he has become engaged in some activity in the playroom. Actually, a perfectly adequate beginning of the evaluation can be carried out with the mother in the room. In fact, in some instances, an unusual opportunity to see the mother-child interaction is provided by such a situation.

As the psychiatrist and child leave to go to *their* room, they are now launched upon a creative venture. No matter how varied the examining psychiatrist's experience has been, this venture will be unique, different in some respects from any other he has had or will have. To be successful, the examination must promise to be a great deal more than a simple fact-finding exploration. Because of the very nature of children, the examining psychiatrist, as a person, will be drawn into a total situation of which both he and the child are parts; later, from this situation he must distill, or abstract, pertinent information that can be applied toward understanding an even larger totality. Harry Stack Sullivan's term *participant observer* is unexcelled as a descriptive phrase—unless we transpose it to *observing participant*.

While the psychiatrist's purpose of seeing the child is the examination, no such perfectly clear idea exists for the child. Younger and more disturbed children make no sharp demarcation between examiner and therapist, parent and adult, or representative of the adult world and extension of the parents. Many children —young and older—may be quite sullen, frightened, angry, or defensive. Thus, the psychiatrist must represent himself as potentially helpful, reasonably open-minded, and comfortably secure in his position, or no process will evolve. Yet, at the same time, he must guard against using this potentially helpful role to rationalize seductiveness, childishness, or blindness to his patient's feelings.

As much pertinent material may be revealed to the psychiatrist during the short walk from the waiting room to the playroom as during his first contact with the family. The child may draw attention to himself by saying, "Isn't this a pretty tie I have on?" Many children will immediately launch into a long and involved fantasy, which they might not bring up later in the play-

room itself; others will even begin discussing events of their life.
Some may try to run off or may "accidentally" trip and hurt or
bump themselves. During this period, the psychiatrist may look for
further reactions to separation from the parents, such as the child's
looking out the window or pointing out the family automobile. This
walk to the office is also an excellent time to observe the typical
posture, coordination, and gait of the child. The psychiatrist will be
unable to make these observations if he is too eager to initiate an
involved conversation that can just as well wait until later.

With the Child

The examining psychiatrist must handle himself with skill
and flexibility, especially during the early interviews with the child.
Once in the playroom, he does not need to instigate or suggest any
particular activity. Let the child take his own tack. He may wish
to look over the toys or to be silent; he may go to work or he may
ask what is going to happen. While in general the psychiatrist
should not impose his own ideas and structure upon the relationship
with his patient until the child has indicated in which direction he
himself intends to move, the psychiatrist must also know when to
move in, when to take the initiative, in order to reassure. Although
the child must have the freedom to determine how close he wishes
to come toward the doctor and at what pace, the psychiatrist must
consider questions of bodily contact and when to allow the child
to approach him. A very sensitive and empathic awareness stands
the psychiatrist in good stead in these issues. For some children,
body contact may come naturally; for others, it can be highly
frightening or seductive. Some children will seek contact with the
psychiatrist as a defensive device or for support; others require
genuinely kind words to help them overcome moments of fright.

In those cases where the child immediately shows unusual
anxiety, the psychiatrist may resort to a timeworn, but often effective, technique by discussing a neutral topic, such as the weather.
Other neutral topics—for example, details of the child's trip to the
clinic—can serve not only as useful icebreakers and a welcome relief
but can easily lead into the child's feelings about the examination
itself. Direct reassurance by giving a simple explanation of his role

as psychiatrist may be helpful for almost all children. For example, in introducing what kind of a doctor he is, the psychiatrist may point out that he is not the type who gives shots. To the anxious child who asks where his mother is, he can answer directly with the added reassurance of a reunion with her at a specific time. Often a young child responds well to being shown on a clock or watch where the "big hand" will be when he can leave to see his mother again.

Special Issues

Children of almost any age are experienced in outwaiting adults. They will try to get the examiner to tip his hand first, sometimes for several interviews. However, aside from allowing an actual panic to develop, the psychiatrist should let the child set the tone and pace of the interview. But the psychiatrist must also be ready to allay undue anxiety by suggesting or initiating activities. And he should not forget that accurate and active interpretation is sometimes by far the most effective means of controlling difficult or anxious behavior. Action—such as holding a child—does not preclude interpretation of the child's fear and rage at the same time.

Often older children will expect (others may specifically try to avoid) some statement of the meaning and purpose of what seems to them a rather strange situation. In the first interview, a very simple and honest statement of the purpose of seeing each child should be made, its precise form depending on the individual psychiatrist. It should include, however, in words suited to the child's age level or assumed level of understanding, an acknowledgment of interest in the child himself—interest in the fact that his parents are concerned enough about him to bring him for an evaluation, and acknowledgment that the evaluative process in many respects will be a partnership.

Usually, the psychiatrist will find it helpful to reintroduce himself to the child or remind him of his name, once in the office. We have here, perhaps, a test of the patient's memory, but, more often, this device serves to restate the psychiatrist's sincere desire to be a real person to the child. It also affords a beginning view of the child's self-awareness and self-concept. After the psychiatrist has mentioned his name again, it follows naturally to ask the child what he himself likes to be called. This question, innocent enough, has the effect of underscoring the individuality of the child, of saying in effect, "I want to take you on your own terms." For instance, parents may persist in calling their son "Billy" when the child would prefer to be called "Bill," or even "William." Hence, some notion of the child's assertiveness and his sense of identity may be gained by his response. If the child insists that he does not care what he is called, the psychiatrist can use the name which feels most natural to him.

Some psychiatrists feel that symptoms which create shame in a child should be mentioned during the first contact. The rationale for broaching the subject is that the child may assume the examiner knows of this symptom. Bedwetting, for example, presents a dilemma. If the topic is not mentioned for some time, the child may assume he is being silently criticized and may then withdraw, and become less and less able to talk. If the psychiatrist senses that the child is withdrawing in such a case he may refer to the symptom early and easily in the process of introducing himself and his job. He may explain that he is the kind of doctor who helps children with certain problems. As he lists common problems —for example, difficulty in school, not getting along well with mother or father, feeling unhappy about one's friends—he can casually include one or two specific symptoms known to bother the child. The success of this technique lies not only in the psychiatrist's attitude toward the symptoms but in his ability to sense when to divert the conversation before the child becomes uncomfortable.

The child's response to this approach provides important data on his attitudes and feelings about his so-called symptoms. Moreover, the examination may, in many cases, demonstrate to the child that help is available for such a symptom as enuresis, or lying, or whatever the symptom happens to be; it follows that some degree of confrontation will be useful. Usually the confrontation is easiest for the child when it occurs in the first contact, or when the groundwork for further discussion is laid in the first contact.

Obviously, generalizations as to procedure can no more be laid down in categorical form than the exploration of an unknown continent can be undertaken from a map. To follow some routine procedure runs the risk of masking material or halting the child's spontaneous expressions and may sometimes even artificially induce anxiety. The best rule is to follow the clues from the material of the child—his behavior, moods, remarks. If the psychiatrist does not follow along with the child, it is impossible for him to gain an adequate view. Children, like adults, will not reveal themselves by force or by following a system. This is equally true in verbally productive older children and in younger children. The problem of the particularly resistive child will be discussed later.

The child should certainly have the opportunity to tell his story in his own way, but whether the psychiatrist focuses on such historical data in the early interviews is problematical. The data may naturally follow from a discussion of the reason for the referral. In gathering this information, the psychiatrist should never sacrifice feelings for the sake of data. He knows he will have the factual information made available by the social worker; besides, his goal is to gain more understanding of the child's feelings, reactions, and struggles in his life situation. In seeking feelings from children, the psychiatrist may find that the direct question, "How did you feel?" may not produce helpful information, especially in latency-aged children. He may get at emotions by asking what a child did about something or what the parent did about something. Here the child's affective response will often become evident.

Before closing the first interview, the psychiatrist will want to give the child a chance to ask any other questions he may have uppermost in his mind. A good method for producing these questions is to discuss factual information on the examination week. The child can be provided with an appointment card of his own, indicating the other examiners he will be seeing during this period. Since the psychiatrist's responsibility is to inform the child of specific examinations, such as laboratory tests, electroencephalograms, and audiometric studies, the conversation over these requirements usually prompts questions. In fact, many individual, as well as fairly usual, reactions will be evoked by this orientation. These reactions, which are also significant in themselves for evaluation purposes, require skillful and understanding handling to allay anxiety. Nevertheless, the psychiatrist should not leave other team members with the undue burden that the child's reaction to their role in the total examination might create. In discussing the psychological testing, the psychiatrist must neither make the child fearful over "taking an exam" nor gloss over the fact that some of the questions will remind him of school tests. It is usually desirable for the psychiatrist to introduce the child personally to the psychologist, though the introduction can be brief. When possible—especially when the child is very anxious—he should also introduce the child to the neurologist.

Confidentiality. Throughout the entire period of the examination the problem of confidentiality of material is present. The first step in the management of any difficulty here lies in the overall attitude of the examining psychiatrist. As discussed in regard to his attitude toward meeting the child, he is the agent of both the child and his parents. He need not trap himself by leaning too far in either direction. Whenever confidentiality becomes an issue, the psychiatrist may look at it as related to the child's conflicts, instead of as a problem of whether or not to divulge information to the parents. Practically speaking, the psychiatrist can assure the child that he will divulge only those things which he feels must be discussed in the child's own best interest; he can also assure him that he will talk over any possible disclosures prior to any discussion. The psychiatrist must consider how the parents may react to certain material. Will they use it destructively? On the other hand, will the information facilitate their understanding of the child's suffering? Suicidal ideas, for example, may well have to be shared, but most of the time a child's confidentiality can be respected by sharing with the parents only general themes of the problems and not specific details. The child may make an issue of confidentiality as a defensive maneuver against deeper understanding of himself and deeper use of the interviews. If the psychiatrist gives too great assurance to the child of confidentiality, this may have the effect of a seductive or even frightening remark. Some children may consider such assurance as an attempt at corruption. After all, the examiner is a new person to the child, who, in spite of his anger with or resentment of his parents, may not feel that he wishes his fate to be entirely in the hands of a stranger. The whole issue requires the psychiatrist's tact and skill and, in general, is best viewed as another potential area for understanding the child and his defensive maneuvers.

Therapeutic Effect. Before ending this discussion on the initial interview, we should look at the therapeutic function of the whole examination. Will the child accept this whole week-long process? Except for rare instances, or perhaps in the initial moments of the first interview, severe negativism seldom interrupts the process if the psychiatrist adopts a generally therapeutic or helpful attitude. Indeed, throughout the week, the skill of the psychiatrist lies in his ability to present himself by nonverbal attitudes, as well as by words, as a potential ally in helping the child manage his own disruptive and pain-producing processes. In so doing, he need not be hampered by too rigid adherence to any artificial distinction between therapy and the examinational process. The examinational process should be therapeutic, if not direct therapy. Even more, it should include at least a sample of what therapy could be like, first, for the purpose of demonstrating such a process to the child, and second, for assessing the child's ability to utilize such a process. In fact, the whole examination should give the general effect of helpfulness; it should demonstrate how an understanding person can be useful, as well as how the process of talking, playing, and interpretive discussion work toward these ends. Hence, in dealing with any initial negativism, the psychiatrist may find it valuable to interpret the child's anger, resentment, or fright. For example, he may discuss with the child his anger and fear at being brought to the clinic. This discussion can be coupled with or followed by both the therapist's acknowledgment that the child's anger is not altogether unjustified and the assertion that the examiner is not necessarily the cause of the evaluation even though he is a party to it. The idea he must convey is that if the child will give him a reasonable chance, he will attempt to understand in an unprejudiced fashion the nature of his problems with his parents, school, or neighborhood.

Beyond the question of the child's overt negativism or reluctance to participate, the central purpose of the examination is to explore all his feelings about himself as a patient. It is not enough to estimate the degree of his disorganization or the extent to which he suffers emotionally. The examination should indicate to what extent he may be capable of introspection; this capacity will vary from child to child. The psychiatrist can judge whether the child can talk about his feelings by showing him examples of important areas of conflict within himself and getting his reactions. Thus, the examination becomes more than the term in the narrow sense implies, because it functions as a medium by which the psychiatrist brings the child's suffering into the open as expressed by unhappiness and defensive and adaptive defenses. The psychiatrist's careful evaluation of the child's reactions to this confrontation turns the examination into a trial therapeutic process.

Practically speaking, the examining psychiatrist should neither be impeded in his exploration by too great a concern with being therapeutic nor held back from being helpful by an overzealous devotion to make his examination "pure." One goal of his examination should be to determine from empirical data as to just which type of psychotherapy (expressive, supportive, psychoanalysis) might benefit the child. In some instances, as the child gains greater awareness of his pain, he himself may be able to see ways toward solution. He may even express a wish for help to his parents directly or symbolically.

INFORMATION

What do we expect to gain from subsequent interviews? The aspects of functioning that the psychiatrist appraises are, of course, reached by inference. Are there special ways to proceed? Are there particular areas of content to cover, even when they are less relevant in some cases than others? How is information gathered for ego strength and defense mechanisms? A few special methods or techniques are available for the collection of data. Nevertheless, we should re-emphasize that the approach to the direct clinical examination of the child is most natural and most effective when the psychiatrist does not feel held to any particular fixed procedure or to an outline that requires an orderly filling in of blanks. The psychiatrist can gain a great deal by following ideas as the child presents them—whether in logical or "psychological" sequence. Furthermore, as the interviews proceed, he receives many new leads from the psychological testing results, the casework process with the parents, and other examinations, including laboratory. Finally, the examiner may sometimes take the initiative and ask the child to discuss specific areas. Opportunities for such questions, if they do not arise naturally, may be made by taking advantage of a lull in the interview. For example, the psychiatrist might frankly say, "You've talked a lot about school, but you haven't told me much about your mother and father," or "Now that you've said a good deal about your father, I wonder whether you could tell me more about your mother." He might even say, "I think I could understand you better if you would tell me about so-and-so."

Some comment about two techniques commonly used may be of interest. These are the three magic wishes and discussion of the child's plans for the future. Both have suffered from being overused and overvalued; as a result, many workers have dropped them as techniques. However, the magic wishes technique in our experience may yield interesting data when viewed in the light of other material. Some deprived children actually wish very directly for material things, such as a bicycle or a million dollars. One eight-year-old boy with a history of epilepsy wished for a million dollars and, in discussing his wish, said he wanted to buy a hospital. Apparently, this indicated his awareness of needing proper care. A child may immediately identify with the examining psychiatrist and wish to become a doctor or a nurse. Some children, rather surprisingly, refer directly to their chief complaint—for example, they may wish for relief from their problem or for a change in their family situation. Often the wishes reflect even greater fantasy. If not overvalued, then a discussion of the child's plans for the future will reveal interesting and helpful information.

Before each meeting with the child, the examiner should review for himself all the previous interviews and the information obtained from the other team members to date. Thus, the psychiatrist prepares himself for the next encounter in much the same way as he prepared himself for the first one. He can anticipate special concerns or material, and he can begin to visualize the general trend that the interviews are taking. He may decide on some area that needs more adequate coverage, speculate on what other information may be valuable, and then, with these ideas in mind, proceed in this direction at the next interview.

The midweek preconference offers a special opportunity—indeed an obligation—for rethinking and making a preliminary summarization. At this time, the examining psychiatrist should have a prepared statement as to his initial diagnostic impressions and tentative recommendations; the degree of finality will vary greatly from family to family. At best, the tentative formulations made at the time of the original planning conference will be either confirmed or corrected at this midweek conference. In some cases, the team may make rather specific plans, such as for testing the reaction of the child (and his parents) to a recommendation for residential treatment, a boarding school placement, or psychotherapy in the home setting. In other instances, the midweek conference may bring into clearer focus the need for continued diagnostic exploration before more specific recommendations can be discussed. The team may consider the need for special examinations—for example, audiometric and neuropsychological studies, additional laboratory studies, and a pneumoencephalogram. The psychiatrist may find it necessary, after the preconference, to pace himself more slowly or, instead, to attempt to speed up his exploration, so that the insights gained from the parents or from the psychological testing of the child may be more effectively correlated with the whole picture. In any event, the results of the preconference will depend upon the somewhat more formal sharing and correlation of material than the team members have experienced earlier in their day-by-day contacts.

Child's Reaction

We sometimes underestimate children's willingness to discuss themselves, their feelings, and their difficulties. Transference and countertransference problems arise. Extremes of countertransference may be reflected in the attitude that the child is either altogether at fault or not at fault at all. Sometimes parents do misunderstand or unjustly misperceive their child's behavior. The examining psychiatrist, by leaning too far backwards to avoid taking the child's side, may, therefore, fail to explore these misperceptions. Here is where the "complaint" does not coincide with the child's true attitude. On the other hand, the psychiatrist may be blinded to his patient's real difficulties when the child tries to present a picture of no concerns or worries. In such instances, the examiner may justifiably ask him why his parents brought him at all. When the child pleads ignorance as to why he was brought to the clinic, the examiner must remember that the child almost always has private thoughts and fantasies about the meaning of the examination. The most realistic and effective position for the examining psychiatrist to take, then, is that, though he understands the child's bewilderment and annoyance over being brought to the clinic, the parents, nevertheless, must have had some reasons for bringing him.

During the evaluation, most children will reveal either directly or symbolically their wish to gain help. For example, if a child knows that a residential unit is attached to the clinic itself, his plea for help may often disguise itself as an interest in the children who live in residence.

Family Setting

To the inferences that the psychiatrist gains from the classical use of play material, such as doll houses, dolls, and other figures, he can add others by exploring the child's living situation. The child's attitude toward siblings, other members of his household, pets, hobbies, community activities, clothes, and material possessions (especially automobiles) are areas for discussion. Many children—when they learn the examining psychiatrist is interested—will talk frankly and enthusiastically about some of the details of their lives, which, in turn, will reflect important aspects of strength and defensive maneuvers.

Although sibling rivalry is often a painful feeling for many children, they can discuss it fairly easily and, in the process, be led to talk about even more painful and difficult material. Often the simple question "Who lives in your house?" opens up conversation about relatives and household help and the child's relationships with them, which the parents have failed either to discuss or emphasize. Similarly, a child's relationship to a pet may present not only an opportunity to empathize with his expression of tenderness, sympathy, or spontaneous pleasure but may also clear the way for gaining his confidence. His pet, likewise, may be a quite useful projection object for unacceptable attitudes in the child himself—for example, the bad puppy who wets in the house.

Discipline and Sexuality

Of course, the more difficult areas of discipline and sexuality are also the business of the examining psychiatrist. Questions about matters for which the child is punished, methods of punishment, and his own attitudes about the fairness of punishment may produce interesting material, as may questions about arguments at home between parents. Such a discussion will probably evoke feelings of disloyalty within the child, which are then grist for the diagnostic mill. The capacity to be an interested but neutral listener can aid the psychiatrist in getting the most out of the child's responses. Questions such as, "Do your parents ever spank you?" or "Do Mother and Father argue a great deal?" may be used. Sometimes the examiner can soften the child's reaction to this kind of questioning by indicating that it is a routine part of the evaluation. Particularly anxious reactions are of significance and may present opportunities for judging the child's reactions to interpretations.

Attitudes toward the body and its processes, sexual information, and masturbation require the psychiatrist to gauge the child's anxiety level carefully. Sexuality is best broached within the context of material that naturally leads into the subject. For example, a sixteen-year-old boy complained that he got no "kick" out of anything. The question "What do you get a kick out of?" allowed a discussion of sexual fantasies. When no opening seems available, questions about sex might be justified on the basis that all children have sexual thoughts and feelings. Although firm reassurance regarding the universality and naturalness of sexual feelings does not remove anxiety, it may allow the child to discuss some of his feelings. Some children may feel free to talk about sex if the psychiatrist asks questions about what their friends say about it, what jokes they tell, and what "dirty" words they use. Another opening for such a discussion may occur—especially for younger children—if the topic of animals' sexual behavior is introduced. For some children—again particularly young ones—the use of colloquial words for sexual organs is more effective, and perhaps even less anxiety provoking, than medical terms. On the other hand, relying on medical terms may be advisable with still other youngsters since it reduces the affective impact. The psychiatrist will, of course, guard against curiosity about sexual matters as an end in itself. To explore sexuality is not a must. The goal in exploring the sexual area is not to find out what the child knows so much as to gain some idea of his attitudes toward sex, his conflicts or anxiety about this area, and the particular pattern his anxieties take, as well as his method of dealing with them.

Outside the Home

Here, again, the child may derive real value from the interest the examiner shows toward his life. Teachers, ministers, Sunday school teachers, and Boy Scout leaders are all meaningful people to the child. His attitudes toward them often reflect not only his relationship with his parents but also reveal important aspects of his relative growth outside the more conflicted home situation. In other words, careful exploration and understanding of the child's adjustment outside the home may reveal that the pathological manifestations in family relationships have not yet incapacitated him to as great an extent as one might expect. On the other hand, a severe degree of disturbance or total incapacitation may be revealed. In the special instance of a so-called school phobia, suffice it to say here that the purpose of the examination may not be to focus predominantly on this symptom. In fact, it may be desirable to avoid such a focus unless the psychiatrist wishes the examination to take clearly and quickly the form of an out-and-out therapy session.

In the areas of church, religious concepts, attitude toward life, and general aspirations there is additional opportunity to explore aspects of the child's conscience, sense of guilt, his conflicts with his parents, and his general attitudes toward authority figures. The degree to which his illness has created a sense of futility and left him unable to think about the future may be gauged. The child's conflicts about identifying with his parents and their attitudes are important areas for exploration. In older children, questions of identity in relation to sexual role confusion may also be studied. Material illuminating a child's self-concepts must be gained from all areas of the examination. The psychiatrist might ask, for example, "Of what are you most proud?" and "What are you most ashamed of in your life?" Answers to these questions are often surprising.

Observations and reports on the child's relations with various people at the clinic can be easily overlooked. However, his approach to secretaries, people in the waiting room, laboratory technicians, and others may present either characteristic or unexpected modes of relating, which shed light on the range of his responses to people who play different roles, and vary as to sex, age, and personality.

Although all phases of the total examination reveal, directly or indirectly, the child's reactions to the psychiatrist, a specific discussion on the examiner as a real person for the child may be helpful. In many respects, the psychiatrist is, of course, a transference figure on whom the child projects many attitudes and feelings. The psychiatrist, as we have said earlier, is also a potential or trial therapist. However, he may function in a third role as a real person who is interested in the child, seemingly understands him, and as a friend or helper can direct him toward gaining help. This last role, if it has been built up during the examination, may also be capitalized on in the final interviews or at the postevaluation conference, at which time the psychiatrist will usually present to the child the same recommendation that he has made to the parents. This is not to say that the psychiatrist will shirk accepting negative responses in presenting the recommendations. Yet, the degree to which he may soften these negative responses so they may be recognized but not openly acknowledged by the child will often depend somewhat on the degree to which he is viewed as a firm, understanding, and clear ally of the patient—an ally who is helping him to master his own difficulties or to recover from his illness.

ORGANIZING DATA

The creative process of understanding, which begins at the moment the child first meets the examining psychiatrist, reaches its climax and summation in the final report on the findings. A succinct outline for the recording and integration of the examinational data is presented by K. Menninger (1962) in *A Manual for Psychiatric Case Study*. A similar outline for drawing the data together on children is given at the end of this chapter.

As discussed earlier, the psychiatrist takes the lead in coordinating and integrating the material of all team members. The data he has obtained in his interviews with the child will never be used independently of other data; in fact, some of the material was evoked during the week in response to information gained from the other disciplines. Nevertheless, the psychiatrist's responsibility is to make his own independent judgment—perhaps it should be called an impression—of the child. He has had the opportunity to clarify, in the midweek preconference, and to test his hypotheses and correct them, in subsequent interviews; as a result, he approaches the final conference with some idea of the eventual outcome. At the conference, where data from the whole week are drawn together from all members of the team, members arrive at both a dynamic assessment of material and an official descriptive diagnosis of the case. A purely running description of the interviews is not a report of the findings, nor is just a description of what seems to be pathological about the child. As emphasized earlier, the whole process of evaluation should reflect the relation of the patient's strengths and assets to his capacity for progress.

We should remember that quite similar neurotic conflicts may be dealt with differently, leading to varying behavioral outcomes. Furthermore, a diagnostic label alone conveys little in many cases. The final report, therefore, should attempt to give a word picture of the child's struggles, his modes of handling them, the relative degree of his success and adaptation, the degree of his suffering, the nature of his awareness of the suffering, and the likelihood of his benefiting from various forms of treatment—including various forms of psychotherapy, temporary hospitalization, or long-term residential treatment. Especially during the final conference the psychiatrist must also think about his findings and recommendations in relation to the parents' personalities, attitudes, and capacity for understanding and using recommendations.

JOINT INTERVIEW

The psychiatrist's job is not completed until he has shared his findings in an interview with the parents and the caseworker. Such an interview occurs immediately after the final staff conference in which the diagnostic impressions and the recommendations are summarized, correlated, and utilized as the specific basis for planning the joint interview with the parents and the caseworker. This interview will not proceed smoothly unless the whole examination week has led to a clear, final integration of all material into usable recommendations, formulated with the parents' resources in mind. The extent to which the examining psychiatrist, as a team member, is clear about both the child's difficulties and the recommendations coming out of the final conference will determine his ease in making a useful presentation at the joint interview. Of course, both the psychiatrist and the caseworker must have a keen appreciation of their roles in order to work comfortably and well together.

At the joint interview, the psychiatrist once again has more than one function. His primary purpose is to present clearly and frankly the team's actual findings on the child to the parents. Understandably, the parents want and expect a reasonably detailed résumé of the findings. Just as understandably, the psychiatrist must be tactful and have the ability to translate technical material into understandable layman's terms. Vague and general comments will not be meaningful, while overly technical remarks will fail to convey truly valuable information to the parents. The psychiatrist's review should include specific references to the physical and neurological examinations, laboratory studies, and the more formal aspects of the child's psychological functioning as determined by the psychological tests. Specific reference to the actual intelligence quotient is avoided for several reasons, one of which is that IQs are often subject to variation—a fact that is hard for parents to understand. While sharing the findings and describing the child's suffering and struggles, the psychiatrist needs to feel, and to exemplify to the parents, an empathy toward their own pain and a concern over their living with the child in his difficulties. Without this empathy, a significant gulf exists between psychiatrist and parents. Recognizing these parental concerns, he should also be able to describe, in an understandable word picture, the sufferings and struggles of the child himself.

The second job of the psychiatrist is to discuss the team's recommendations to the parents. This presentation should not be rushed and ideally should follow naturally upon the findings. On occasion, the parents will have some idea of what the recommendations will be if the findings have been presented clearly, carefully, and with empathy. Generally, however, the psychiatrist should not expect the parents to agree to the recommendations too readily. Inevitably, they will have many reactions and feelings; as a result, these have to be worked through before the recommendations can occur. Such a process must continue within the context of the relationship the parents have developed with the caseworker throughout the week of examination. Thus, the psychiatrist will wish to refer many of the questions and feelings about the recommendations to the caseworker while he is still in the interview room. Before he leaves, the psychiatrist, in fact, may try to set the stage for continued discussion.

Keeping in mind his considerations in regard to goals of the joint interview with the parents we can add a few notes on the psychiatrist's way of proceeding. In most instances, he will find it helpful to open his discussion by asking both parents what is now uppermost in their minds. This focus makes the findings more meaningful and allows the sharing of findings to follow more naturally from the concerns of the parents. It contributes to better understanding of any divergent reactions they may have. If either parent remains relatively silent, the psychiatrist can direct questions to the less active one. He must use careful judgment in directing a question to the caseworker; but he must be alert to the need for the caseworker to enter the discussion when one or both parents show anxiety.

The timing of the psychiatrist's departure from the room should be based mainly on his judgment of the degree to which the parents seem to be shifting from a review of the findings to expressing their feelings about the recommendations. Usually, he will have to take the initiative for his departure; thus, he may specify openly that the parents will probably wish to discuss the issues further with the caseworker. To remain until the parents seem completely comfortable is a mistake. The psychiatrist may even specify that the parents should discuss their feelings within the context of their talks with the caseworker during the week.

SHARING FINDINGS

In most instances, a crucial part of the examination process comes when the psychiatrist discusses the findings with his patient. Perhaps, if the child is very young and quite disturbed, such a discussion is best omitted. As with the parents, the opening remarks are those that relate to areas closest to the child. In reviewing the recommendations, the psychiatrist may use material he has uncovered and discussed with his patient during the previous interviews. This approach helps to make them meaningful to the child, even if the child's immediate response is negative. When desirable he may refer to the parents' wish that the child gain help, so he will not continue to be so unhappy. The psychiatrist, as bearer of the team's findings, must stand ready to be the recipient of much anger and to accept it without any other reaction than recognizing it with the child. He may use examples of the child's contacts with specialists at the clinic as illustrations of the kind of help he may get from another doctor. He may sometimes help the child with separation fears. He also has the opportunity to dispel possible misconceptions about being "crazy" or being "put away." He can then terminate this final meeting with some expression of pleasure in having seen the child and some hope for the child's future happiness.

We cannot close without some reference to reports by other psychiatrists on the examination of the child. This examination in many respects is an individualized process, and it is impossible to separate completely the examination of the child from the total diagnostic study of the family by a diagnostic team or from the more formal psychological study that, in part, utilizes psychological testing. Levy's (1929) article—a classic in the field—is so very helpful in its discussion of the physical examination that it is virtually essential reading for all members of a team. Chess (1959), Finch (1960), Harrison and Carek (1966), Kanner (1957), Kessler (1966), and Pearson (1949) will also be of particular interest to the reader in gaining a broader perspective on the examinational and diagnostic process.

OUTLINE FOR CASE SUMMARY

I. Administrative data

Child's full name, age, birthdate (in parentheses), sex, order of birth in respect to siblings, name, and hometown of the parents, father's and mother's occupations, nationality, and parents' marital status. Names of brothers and sisters may be included, if desired, as well as other pertinent information, such as adoption, and child's grade in school. An example making use of this approach is as follows: John Doe, age nine (birthdate: 6–1–60), is the second of five children and the oldest of two sons of Mr. and Mrs. John Doe, Sr., of 2221 West Sixth Street, Topeka, Kansas. Mr. Doe is a lawyer; Mrs. Doe is a schoolteacher. The other children are Mary, age eleven, Peter, age seven, Jody, age four, and Ann, age two.

Next, state the source and location of referral but do *not* mention the reason for referral. Then, give the beginning and ending date of the examination, and state explicitly whether both parents participated, and, if so, how long. In a separate paragraph add the following sentence: *This is a confidential case summary for professional use only, and is under no circumstances to be shown to any member of the family.*

II. Clinical data

A. Historical data

1. The chief complaint: State here the symptom or symptoms as first observed, or the reason for referral, or the

reason for the initiation of the psychiatric case study. From here on, any reference to time should be in terms of the patient's age, as well as the date of the event.

2. Background: Start with an extremely short, objective description of the father's and mother's physical appearance and demeanor, including their age. Briefly describe pertinent data from the parents' childhoods and backgrounds, give their marital history, and the relationship of the marital interaction as it is specifically related to the child. However, do not, at this point, discuss any of the casework data. If there are other siblings, state briefly their level of mental health.

Then summarize those factors in the pregnancy, birth, infancy and childhood development, schooling, sexual and social behavior, and purely medical history that are pertinent to the understanding of the child and to the diagnosis. Events and their sequences along with the reactions of the child and his parents to these events should be included. Previous examinational data, if relevant, should be reviewed unless these would fall more logically under the heading of "Present Illness" or "Examinational Data." Also mention family history and factors related to siblings if they have importance for the case.

3. Present illness: Describe the major events and developments, including the more important symptoms, leading up to the present examination. Explain what seems to have been the family's immediate reason for coming at this time.

B. Examinational data

1. Physical examination: Give the date and be sure to mention height, weight, and pubertal status, if relevant. Describe only significant findings.

2. Neurological examination (if applicable): Give the date and describe all the pathological findings and the strengths observed in the neurological examination,

based on the neurologist's report. Do not just use the summary at the end of his report, which frequently does not repeat such important items as observed "soft" neurological signs. End this paragraph with the neurologist's conclusions, beginning the sentence with "Neurological Impression."

3. Laboratory examinations (as applicable): Give the dates. Describe the lab tests and X-rays. Specify X-ray of wrists for bone age. If the electroencephalogram is abnormal, briefly describe the abnormalities and do not give just the electroencephalographer's final opinion.

4. Psychiatric examination: In one or two paragraphs, state the findings from the psychiatric examination, beginning with the number of hours spent with the child. The first sentence may begin thus: "In the psychiatric examination, which consisted of five interviews." Try to organize your findings of the patient as a meaningful whole, rather than making it a checklist of the psychological outline.

Follow these paragraphs with a summary of the psychological tests, which may start as follows: "In the psychological testing situation" or "From the psychological tests." Do not use the summary of the tests that the psychologist prepared in his report, as it may not contain the test data most pertinent to the final picture. Instead, take the most significant findings from the test report and always include the intelligence quotient; mention the test on which this IQ was obtained and its relation to previous quotients, factors affecting the test, and important qualifications—such as the fact that in this case the IQ is simply the average of widely varying scores on different functions. It may be useful to specify the areas of best and poorest functioning.

If signs of organic impairment are found, explain what these signs are, without going into too much detail. Mention such things as distortions in visual perception, difficulty in eye-hand coordination, gross motor co-ordination, and so on. At the end, list all the tests that were given to the patient.

Note: The examinations referred to and summarized above are usually those made by the reporting examiners. If the summary is made after re-evaluation of the child, the examinational data from the previous examination may be discussed under "Examinational Data," or it can be included under the headings of "Background" and "Present Illness," whichever will be most useful.

5. Speech and hearing examination: State the findings of the speech pathologist here. If no examination has been performed, simply omit this heading.

6. Reports of other examinations: State the findings of any special examinations, such as those done by the neuro-psychologist, pediatrician, or other medical specialists.

C. Observational data: Discuss changes observed in the child during the examination, if any. Then, in the next paragraph, discuss the casework with the parents, beginning the paragraph in the following manner: "In the casework process with the parents." Discuss here the changes which occurred in each parent's attitudes, feelings, and opinions. Describe how the parents came to grips with the casework process (or whether they did not), their relationship with the caseworker, and their use of the relationship to examine attitudes and feelings. If the findings were discussed with the parents in casework prior to the final conference, a description of their reaction to the findings can be given, but their reaction to the recommendations should be left for later in the summary, and a description of the case-work should be carried up to the point of the final con-ference only. Do not refer to the worker; merely give the parents' reactions. Finally, in another paragraph, discuss any changes occurring in the parent-child interaction during the examination.

III. Diagnostic and prognostic conclusions
    A. Appraisal of the environment

Give here the child's "social diagnosis," including the family constellation, the family's cultural and socioeconomic status, as well as any special environmental difficulties, such as school adjustment and legal troubles.

B. Appraisal of the patient
  1. Somatic structure, functions, and reactions:
    a. Give here the child's special assets (physical, psychological, and neurological assets of psychological significance).
    b. Impairment: Here are given official medical and neurological diagnoses, with dates.
  2. Psychological structure, functions, and reactions:
    a. Give here the child's assets and potentialities (sublimations, talents, intelligence, sensitivity, insight, positive aspects of his ways of struggling with or compensating for difficulties, and so forth).
    b. His impairments and liabilities, which include the following:
      (1) Preclinical disorganization: A brief statement should be made as to the patient's predisposition to the present illness, related to congenital factors, pregnancy or birth difficulties, early infantile problems of achieving an equilibrium, and so forth, pre-existing personality disorders, disabilities, and the adaptational obstacles they presented.
      (2) Present disorganization:
        Degree: Mild, moderate, severe.
        Type: Acute, chronic, episodic, recurrent.
        Trend: Stationary, increasing, decreasing; rapid, slow, variable.
        Syndrome: Give the most nearly appropriate APA designation, including code number.
        Symptoms and signs: List main features on which above diagnosis is based.

C. Explanatory formulation
  This is the place to discuss such aspects of the case as the

genetic, developmental, and dynamic understanding of the child's difficulties and the dynamics of the interaction between the parents and the child, as they were formulated in the final conference by the team.

D. Prognosis

Probabilities regarding the further trend of disorganization with and without therapeutic intervention should be stated, with time estimates. Accessibility of the patient to treatment (motivation, cooperation, and financial situation of the family should also be indicated). If outpatient treatment is recommended, mention possibilities of favorably changing the home environment. If continued case study is desirable, state this here, along with what it will take and the time involved before a clearer diagnostic understanding can be reached.

IV. Treatment recommendations

If any recommendations were made for any kind of somatic therapy—for example, medications—enumerate them in the first paragraph, stating also who will be responsible for the treatment, if this is known.

Then, in the following paragraph, discuss recommendations for psychological therapy, and the type, including residential treatment, psychotherapy, and remedial treatment—for example, remedial reading. Do not mention any specific treatment centers, but merely describe in general what you have in mind. Be sure also to mention whether future casework with the parents was recommended.

V. Addenda

A. Final conference with the parents

Discuss here the parents' reactions to the findings and recommendations, along with their further plans. Mention factors which may prevent, limit, or impel the carrying out of these recommendations and what, if any, assistance the parents will need in carrying out the recommendations. State also from whom these assistance measures are necessary and to whom the parents have been referred for this step.

B. Further follow-up information

This heading is optional and should be used only where time has elapsed between preparation of the summary and the end of the examination, and if there is anything to add that will have significance. This information would include subsequent developments, responses, complications, new information about the patient or environment, or radical changes in the external situation.

HAPTER $V\!I\!I\!I$

The Role of
Conferences

W_e have seen that our clinic's major goal in
an intensive psychiatric assessment of a patient is to provide a
clinical process in which both parents and child participate. This
process, which is multidisciplinary in approach, attempts to gather
information in such a way that the clinical team can arrive at a
sound formulation from which to make meaningful and realistic
recommendations. At the same time—and neither divorced from

216

nor independent of the findings and recommendations—the examination should also provide a process through which the child's parents can gradually accept and understand the findings and thus act positively toward the recommendations.

In order to approximate such goals, particularly in the relatively short examination period of five days, it is necessary to evolve a broad conference structure that points toward optimum communication among the team members and integrates their separate but related efforts. The mainstays of this structure are three conferences set within the timespan of the examination. The one-hour planning conference takes place two days before the first actual contact with the child and his family. The one-hour preconference takes place on the morning of the third day of the examination process. A two-hour final conference takes place on the fifth day of the procedure. These conferences have two major functions: the first function is oriented toward the goals of assessment (clinical function) and the second is oriented toward the training and experience (training function). The reader has already had an introductory glimpse of some of the clinical functions as seen by the social worker, by the psychologist, and by the psychiatrist. In this chapter we will look at the conferences in relation to each other and to the total process.

CLINICAL FUNCTION

In order to begin to think about the different functions of the planning conference, the preconference, and the final conference, as well as the peculiarities of all three, we might consider them against the backdrop of a nonexistent "easy" examination. Let us assume an imaginary situation in which the child and his parents were referred to the clinic by their family physician. All the family accepted the referral with ease, all the referral material was sent to us promptly upon request, and all the necessary arrangements for the examination were made smoothly and efficiently. The parents cooperated further by sending a sequence of pictures of the child from the time of birth, and each parent sent his own version of the child's medical, developmental, social, and academic history. The planning conference was held two days before the beginning

of the examination and the team agreed that no additional information was necessary. Members also agreed as to why the child was
being brought to the clinic at that particular time and what the
parents and child wanted to obtain from the examination. In addition, the team agreed as to the probable diagnostic implications and
the general areas of difficulty predictable within the examination
process.

The parents and the child arrived on schedule, and the
mother and father were able to work freely and comfortably in
their relationship with the psychiatric social worker from the very
beginning. The child was also able to work well with the child
psychiatrist and the child psychologist during the first and second
days of the examination. On the morning of the third day of the
examination, the preconference was held and the high points of the
pertinent referral material were quickly reviewed; all three members
of the team shared the clinical findings with one another and their
conference leader, and those supervisors who elected to be present.
Preliminary reports from the neurologist and the speech pathologist
were also shared. By now, the clinical picture was beginning to
emerge from the referral material and from the new clinical contacts and data. The task of each team member for the remainder
of the examination was fairly clear. Throughout that time the team
continued to be in close communication, and by virtue of this contact and the integration of the clinical material, the diagnostic
picture became sufficiently clear for the psychiatric social worker
to begin to discuss the tentative diagnostic findings with the parents
and also to discuss possible recommendations with them and to
explore their reactions.

By the afternoon of the fifth day of the examination, the
picture had continued to unfold, and all three team members were
in complete harmony as to the findings and recommendations to
be made. Each one brought to the final conference well-prepared
summaries of his contribution to the evaluation process. During the
first part of the conference, all this material was presented along
with that of the neurologist and the speech pathologist, as well as
the findings from the roentgenological and encephalographic labora-
tories. During the second hour of the conference, these findings and

the recommendations were discussed and elaborated by the team, the conference leader, and the other staff members present. At the final conference everyone concurred with the team's findings and recommendations, and the evaluation was concluded by postconference interviews; the psychiatric social worker and the child psychiatrist met with the parents, and the child psychiatrist met with the child. The parents were able to accept both the findings and the recommendations and were ready to start implementing the latter.

Even though the above example is probably an impossible ideal, it does help to represent in a rather simple and transparent way how the conferences should relate to and function as a part of the total process of assessing a child within his family. Each of the participating disciplines contributes the direct-contact parts of the assessment; these, along with special consultations and laboratory findings, must continuously undergo integration. As a result, the outcome will be as meaningful as possible and useful findings and recommendations, rather than a simple sum of information, will emerge. Conferences, then, are special integrating techniques, catalysts as well as clarifiers of an unfolding process. They are a special device for communication among team members, as compared with ordinary and continual communication that team members share throughout the examination process. Conferences are also a special kind of break in an unfolding examination. They are time-breaks during which each participant examines and re-examines his own material along with that of his co-workers from his own point of reference; they are time-breaks in which the team members bring their findings and interpretations of those findings to sharper examination by sharing them and discussing them with each other, as well as with their other peers and colleagues.

PLANNING CONFERENCE

Often a great deal of information and data are available to the clinical team prior to the actual beginning of the examination. In many instances, parents bring their child from several hundreds of miles away, and their arrival is almost always preceded by considerable correspondence. Quite often, children are referred after having had a variety of earlier psychiatric examinations and treatment experiences. Many of the children have been in special educational programs, and the parents may have been in psychiatric treatment or in casework because of their child's difficulties. We noted earlier that as much pertinent information as possible is obtained before the actual start of the examination. When the child is referred from our own local area, referral information is most often augmented by the parents' participation in an interview with the caseworker prior to the examination, while the child is usually seen in psychiatric consultation.

Before the assigned clinical team meets a child and his parents, each member must carefully sift through, weigh, evaluate, and absorb the considerable information available from his own particular point of reference. After having studied and digested these data, the team members meet with the assigned senior psychiatrist conference leader two days before the beginning of the examination in order to discuss their tentative formulations. These discussions involve not only their impressions as to the kind of clinical problems involved in the case but also the family's early attitudes, motivations, and expectations in regard to the examination, along with their possible reactions to various aspects of the examination once it has gotten under way. Also discussed are the special traps, pitfalls, and other areas of technical difficulty that individual team members in all probability will have to face. Actual arrangements regarding the first day of the examination may also be discussed. For example, from the preliminary material a decision usually must be made as to whether or not the first hour of the examination should include the parents, the social worker, the child, and the child psychiatrist in one group.

PRELIMINARY CONFERENCE

On the morning of the third day of the examination, the team, their supervisors, and the conference leader meet for a preconference. Each team member's individual examination work has been going on for two days, during which time he has repeatedly communicated with the others about their part of the examination. The tasks of the preconference are complex and multifaceted and grow out of the presentation of the material by each member and out of its discussion by the total team. Each attempts to bring what he, as a member of a particular discipline and as a specific individual, has been able to learn about the child and about the family interaction. Each brings his material as a direct contribution to the evaluation and also adds indirectly by contributing to the understanding of the other individuals and disciplines involved. Individual contributions tend to clarify the puzzling aspects of other team members' findings. Each member attempts to bring into more meaningful focus the referral material, the tentative formulations based on this, the first findings at this clinic, and the preliminary diagnostic findings and recommendations. Useful integration of this material comes through free and constructive discussion of it. In our setting we believe that this is best accomplished by having the conference chaired by a senior staff psychiatrist who is not directly participating in the study and by having the team supervisors participate in the conference, particularly when the team members are trainees. In its function of coordinating and integrating clinical findings and efforts, the preconference not only gives focus to the clinical picture as it exists at the moment but, in the process, illuminates which aspects of the pre-examination and referral material are validated and which need supportive data. The conference points out disagreements within all the data and raises appropriate questions as to their meanings. The preconference thus tests and challenges the preconceptions underlying the first views of the case and then revises them.

The preconference reveals the extent to which the total examination actually is an integrated and unfolding process. Even more dramatically, it indicates when the work is not developing in a constructive way. The preconference can then usually provide the information and intelligence by which the situation may be remedied. An example of such a problem exists in the situation in which a rather strong apparent or actual divergence of opinion exists initially among team members in their emerging impressions of a child's difficulties. Most often during the preconference itself, the elaboration of the seeming differences usually results in a larger mutual understanding and agreement.

The preconference also serves the function of preventing,

revealing, and tentatively resolving the destructiveness of discordant forces that may be at work or develop prior to or during an examination. These may arise from transference or countertransference feelings that are at least latent in any clinical interaction. The work and the orientation of the preconference also mitigate against personal disagreements and struggles within the clinical team. These can emerge out of personality clashes unrelated to the evaluation as such, as well as out of countertransference distortions.

FINAL CONFERENCE

The final conference is a special time-break near the very end of the examination process. As such, it has all of the functions of the preconference, with an emphasis on certain tasks which have developed because the data gathering and actual examinational parts of the total assessment procedures have been completed. In one sense, the final conference is a clinical afterthought. The clinical contact with the child and his parents is all but over, except for the postconference interviews. Each team member has already collected, analyzed, and interpreted his data. Yet, in a more important sense, the final conference is not an afterthought at all but a vital and a most important segment of the whole process, out of which emerges the essence of the total effort. Again, each team member brings in, for shared study, understanding, interpretation, and integration into a broader understanding, all his clinical findings and his interpretation of any recommendations relative to them. Out of this information, along with the laboratory reports and the findings of special consultants, the conference must derive specific as well as broad understandings of the child and his particular environment, and the interrelated needs of both.

As to be expected, the nature of the final conference is highly dependent upon everything that has preceded it in the examination. It is possible—at least theoretically as our example showed earlier—to have a clinical evaluation proceed so smoothly and be so well integrated and intelligible as to preclude the necessity for a formal final conference. This simple illustration, which delineated the relationship of the conference to the total evaluation process, also indicated that the more nearly the ideal of a smooth, continuously integrated process is approached, the more nearly the final conference is a flowing continuation of the preconference. When this does not occur, the major task of reaching a clear understanding of the clinical problem remains for the final conference. When the reflection upon the clinical findings and their integration are left as a task for the final conference, the psychiatric social worker's work with the parents is limited as is the psychiatrist's work with the child. They are not able to begin discussion of possible findings and recommendations before the final conference if a tentative agreement has not emerged from earlier discussion. The less the psychiatrist has been able to help them understand and accept the clinical findings and the recommendations, the less he will be able to help them respond constructively toward implementing the recommendations. Little or nothing positive can happen if recommendations based on an absolutely valid clinical picture of the child and his family are met by immobility resulting from incomplete acceptance on the part of the parents.

The format of the final conference is the same as that of the preconference. The content of a conference ranges all the way from extremely clear, well-ordered presentations by the team members—presentations from which the findings and recommendations readily evolve to find complete acceptance—to presentations of material from which the findings and recommendations must be sifted, threshed, and sieved by spirited, sometimes heated, and often weighty discussions.

The participating pattern for the final clinic conference is almost exactly the same as the one described for the preconference. The usual clinical team, along with the neurologist and the speech pathologist, makes presentations. Each presentation is written out ahead of time to insure that it is inclusive, concise, pertinent, and well organized. As the result of such thoughtful planning, the second half of the conference remains for the rest of the work to be done. The conference is supervised by a senior staff member who has not been directly involved in the clinical examination but has supervised the earlier conferences. His role varies and may include listening, questioning, facilitating, teaching, discussing, playing the devil's advocate, calling on specific individuals, protecting the floor for a particular contributor, watching the time, keeping or changing the focus, and—when necessity demands it—even making an arbitrary decision.

Senior staff members who may be called on by the chairman or the other conferees may also participate in the final conference as consultants. In fact, all may participate actively or passively in the conference. When necessary, certain staff members are particularly requested to attend. Appropriate visitors are also welcome to attend the final conference, but an attempt is made to keep their number at any particular conference small in proportion to the total number of participants, so as not to alter the character of the proceedings too much. Too many visitors can interfere with the work of a conference, even though they do not actually contribute.

TRAINING FUNCTION

Case conferences not only contribute to the clinical work at hand but also have very important training functions. In the sense that experience can be a good teacher, every person present at a clinical conference has an opportunity to learn, regardless of whether or not he participates. Active participation through making a presentation, acting as supervisor, or taking part in the discussion, increases the training potential. Participation by several supervisors results in a group interaction among them which adds breadth and depth to the training regularly provided by individual supervision.

There are no property boundaries related to the availability of conference material for learning or teaching. Thus, all disciplines should be involved in case conferences and individuals at all levels of training and experience should attend. Such attendance is of great importance in a clinical setting that supports a training program in psychiatric social work, child psychology, and child psychiatry, as compared with a setting that has a training program for only one discipline.

In addition to their clinical function, case conferences must spell out for participants the basis and rationale upon which diagnosis, treatment plan, and prognosis are derived; these are clearly essential for the purpose of thorough training. This is one more reason why a truly meaningful conference does not dare to be a production staged by the responsible clinical team for a captive audience. There is no audience. Every person present should regard himself as a member of the conference, even the silent visitors. Also, clinical function and training function must not be separated. However, the excellent teaching potential of a certain aspect in a case must not take up so much time and emphasis that meeting the responsibilities of the actual clinical problem is endangered. Thus, the conference leader must protect and determine the balance.

In a broader sense, case conferences have yet another training function. Since these conferences delineate the role and the function of each team member, they might be called the exhibit case of the clinical team. They illustrate the integrative, supplementary, and complementary way in which the various disciplines are able to interact toward a common goal. This process is not necessarily self-perpetuating, so all staff members must pay close attention in order that it may be understood, learned, and successfully continued.

In a still broader sense, case conferences are also the showcase, or even the benchmarks of a given clinical setting. Conferences reflect orientation and philosophy in a very direct and concrete way. They reflect the meaning of "clinical team" at a particular clinic. And they clearly reflect the way in which each participating discipline makes its own unique contribution, as well as the way in which each is valued.

~~~~~~

CHAPTER IX

Team Function and Misfunction

~~~~~~

We have seen that the diagnostic process of the clinical team, stressed earlier (Chapter Eight), involves a constant sharing and integration of contributions from the different disciplines. It is an evolving synthesis, not just a final adding up; to achieve this synthesis requires continuous interchange among the team members. Information from one discipline will be used in the process of another, and hypotheses that might appear valid from the limited perspective of a particular discipline may be found to be invalid when viewed from the broader context of the total process.

It is, of course, difficult to discuss adequately such a complex interaction briefly; thus, questions of which aspects to stress and which to neglect have to be rather arbitrarily decided. We first illustrate the interdisciplinary process with a case example typical of a number of controversial problems brought to the clinic.* Then we consider some complications which may arise in this process, especially those problems which may occur when inexperienced members first join the team. Such an emphasis may help to acquaint workers new to the field with some of the potential difficulties; hopefully, out of this awareness, some problems can be avoided or more easily resolved.

In our brief review of a case process, it is impractical to include the total record. Many details of the workers' processes with the parents and child have to be omitted or summarized very briefly. This is unfortunate, because steps in the process may then seem unclear. For instance, in our first case illustration, major progress occurred in the parents, but since we cannot include much of the social work process, there is not enough evidence of how this change took place. Similar difficulties arise in trying to describe the backstage interaction among the team members, since only selected samples of this interaction can be included.

In the case illustration that we will present, we will describe our usual way of working; we recognize that this approach is geared to our own special situation and need and that some features may not be best for other child psychiatry settings. As a matter of fact, we have no rigid, completely standard way of proceeding, as this must be flexible in order to adapt to the needs of each case. Moreover, in the process of evolution new approaches are tried and old ones are dropped when their usefulness has been outgrown. For instance, since this case was recorded, a speech pathologist and a neuropsychologist have been added to the diagnos-

---

* Some of the material used has been obtained by an "observer" following a series of outpatient evaluations, recording both the scheduled and the more spontaneous contacts among the various team members.

tic team, and a planning conference of the members is regularly scheduled to review advance information on the parents and child before they arrive at the clinic. Although each case and each team process are unique and have certain characteristics all their own, there are nevertheless certain general principles common to all. In the particular case selected, the following features make it useful to illustrate some of these principles:

1. The case presents a somewhat common and relatively uncomplicated diagnostic problem, even though a full study had never before been undertaken; in previous clinical contacts, only fragments of the total problem had been considered.

2. The case demonstrates the use of the interdisciplinary team in obtaining all the pertinent information and shows how this is used to help the family.

3. The case illustrates that, although the team members involved were both inexperienced in working with each other and relatively new to the field, through mutual cooperation and the assistance of supervisors and team leaders, they were able to achieve a relatively successful process.

4. The case indicates how parents sometimes find it easier to understand and accept undisputed cerebral palsy or unquestionable retardation than scattered deficits, which are further complicated by the child's defensive response to frustration. This case also shows both how careful the team has to be to avoid getting involved in previous experts' disagreements and how patient the members must learn to be with frustrated, confused, and difficult parents.

CASE ILLUSTRATION

Background: Mr. and Mrs. G. requested an evaluation of their youngest son, Harold, age nine and a half, because they had been given two conflicting professional opinions about the causes of his severe learning difficulties. One opinion was from the boy's private tutor, who felt Harold had an emotional block and, therefore, could not learn. This emotional block he believed was related to the boy's extreme dependency on his mother. As a result, the tutor believed, the boy needed to be immediately separated from his parents and have treatment in a residential center. He stated that, in early tutoring sessions, Harold's hyperactivity and constant head movement suggested possible brain damage, but as a positive relationship developed between tutor and pupil, the movements decreased. He administered the Stanford-Binet, Form L, and the boy obtained an IQ of 92. The tutor felt his actual IQ was somewhat higher but that his tension and anxiety during the testing and his overall emotional disturbance affected the score. A differing opinion was held by the psychologist who had twice tested Harold. He reported a history of slowness and said that in testing the boy a year apart with the Revised Stanford-Binet, he found the boy had IQ scores of 85 and 84. The psychologist further stated that although there was evidence of personality difficulties and that although psychotherapeutic help would certainly be worth while, he did not feel as radical a plan as recommended by the tutor was indicated—especially since the school principal reported that Harold's present social adjustment was not too poor and the parents felt he was improving both socially and emotionally.

Before contacting the Menninger Clinic, the parents had also tried to obtain help from two agencies but felt they had gotten nowhere in these efforts. Obviously, they were not demanding that we assume the role of arbitrators; at the same time they made it clear that they were ready to fight us should be we critical of them or report findings that they did not want to hear. Before the actual evaluation, through a series of telephone calls and letters, the coordinator of examinations explored further the parents' motivations for coming to the clinic and acquainted them with the nature of the experience they would have here. Thus, considerable preliminary work was done before the family arrived, and considerable information about them was already available to the team.

Family and Team Interaction: On the first morning, the coordinator of examinations, the team social worker, and the team psychiatrist were in the staff room, going over the case material. When the family arrived, the coordinator, who had handled the communications with the family, introduced himself to them and then introduced the social worker and psychiatrist. The boy then went with the psychiatrist, while the parents went to a conference with the social worker. (Although joint interviews of parents and child with the psychiatrist and social worker are also often useful, they were not used in this case.)

After their interviews with Harold and his parents, the social worker and the psychiatrist met to share their initial impressions. The social worker reported:

Mr. G. appears to be negativistic, angry, and indignant, while his wife looks tired, tense, and troubled in a sad sort of way. I immediately got the impression of two people in separate camps, facing each other like enemies, one challenging the rights of the other. Neither seems aware of their mutual struggle over the boy. Mrs. G. said the child has always been slow and was born with a club foot, which was a great shock to her. She feels the boy has always demanded a great deal of help. In a challenging, hostile manner, Mr. G. indicated that Harold is too dependent on his mother. He threateningly announced that he is a domineering, headstrong man who feels he can handle his son if he were only given the chance. Almost with bravado, he firmly said that unless separation from the child is terribly vital, he will not consider it, since he can do more for Harold than anyone else. I felt a smouldering anger in Mrs. G. as she was being attacked by her husband, but she didn't defend herself, except to restate in a rather lame way that Harold had been slow in walking, talking, and learning many things. Mr. G. made it clear before the end of the hour that since he and his wife do not view the problem in the same way, they want us to decide their course of action. "Tell us," he said, "what is wrong with the boy and give us a *firm* recommendation. We'll do our best to follow it if we can."

The psychiatrist then offered the social worker his impression that the child, in addition to his retardation, showed other evidences of brain damage—for instance, his difficulties in the perceptual-motor area:

He shows poor coordination and is generally awkward. On two occasions he lost his balance and fell on the stairs. While getting a drink of water, he twice dropped the paper cup after filling it with considerable difficulty. In addition, he has perceptual difficulties. He attempted to fit a large square block into a smaller round hole, trying two or three times to get them to fit. He finally gave up from frustration, not because he actually "saw" the discrepancy in size and shape.

After giving further details, the psychiatrist wondered whether the parents showed any awareness that the child was brain-damaged. The social worker told him that they seemed unaware, though they did feel the boy was somewhat slower than other children. What they stressed was their confusion, as they had been given conflicting professional advice in the past as to whether the child needed placement. They admitted that they did not know how to resolve this problem. "We want to find out," they said, "whether our son is emotionally blocked and what we can do to help him." Although the mother gave the impression of wanting to consider placement of the child, the social worker thought the father would need considerable help if the clinic suggested the child should be separated from the home. In spite of calling himself impatient and short-tempered, the father was so emotionally involved that he was toying with the idea of working part time, so he could spend a few more hours with his son; this sacrifice seemed to be tied in with his feeling that he had to prove to himself that he was adequate as a father. At the same time, the social worker wondered about his statement that his business took him out so much in the evening that he was unable to be with the child, whose care was then up to the mother. She questioned whether he needed to be out that much; his business involvement might be a way to avoid sharing the difficulties in looking after his son.

The social worker also had the tentative impression that the father almost needed to be led by the hand and have someone confirm that what he was doing was right; she had even had to help him with suggestions about what to tell the child about his being at the clinic. She reported the father had told his son only that they were coming here on business. The team psychiatrist also confirmed that this was what Harold had told him. The social worker then went on to say that the mother had emphasized how demanding she felt the child to be; she also believed she was overprotective and too indulgent, blaming this behavior on Harold's club foot and need for special care.

The team psychiatrist considered this information in relation to the extremely difficult, demanding way the boy had responded to him and said, "He became progressively more anxious, restless, and dissatisfied. He was provocative and ordered me about, demanding that I do things for him and becoming very angry and irritable if I refused. He was also fearful and once tried to return to his mother. He refused to talk about this behavior, and any direct questions I asked met with 'I don't know' or 'I won't tell you.' " The psychiatrist speculated on what it would be like to live with such a child. The social worker told him that the child apparently noticed the parents' irritation with him, because they reported he often said before beginning his incessant questioning, "I want to ask you something but please don't be angry."

From this interchange, the social worker knew that he had to explore further why the parents—particularly the father—needed to deny to a large extent the child's probable handicaps and limitations. She also had a tentative impression of the child from the psychiatrist that she could compare with the parents' picture of the child; in turn, she had given the psychiatrist her impression of the parents with which he could compare the impression he received from the boy. The psychiatrist also realized that since the parents did not view the child as he did, he would have to make a careful study of the evidence for brain damage and retardation, so he could explain the discrepancy in viewpoints. Having learned from the boy of Harold's fear of his parents' anger and impatience, he knew that both he and the social worker would have to investigate how much this fear was realistically based on the parents' behavior with their son and how much of it was an exaggerated concern on the part of the boy. The psychiatrist had also obtained confirmation of the child's statement that the parents had been unable to tell him the real reason for bringing him to the clinic. This was another indication of the parents' fearfulness, which had to be explored further. Thus, from their conversation, both the social worker and the psychiatrist had learned something of the nature of the problems each faced in his individual processes. They had also confirmed some aspects of the reports from those who had previously seen the child —for example, his dependency on the mother—and they had found further evidence of the possibility of brain damage, which, though mentioned in the referring reports, had been insufficiently explored.

On the first day of the diagnostic examination, the team

psychiatrist also sought out the team psychologist to tell him the boy might be resistive and hyperactive. He shared with the psychologist, too, the evidence he had for his impression of brain damage and intellectual retardation, and described his difficulties with the boy. Later, during the day, all the team members happened to be in the general meeting room at the same time, and the psychologist stated that although he had been expecting difficulty, he found instead that the boy behaved "like an angel." He suggested to the team psychiatrist that with a more organized, structured approach he might also see different behavior. The psychologist then reported that on the tests he had given so far, the boy appeared to be quite limited intellectually. Before the meeting ended, the social worker also briefly repeated to the psychologist her impressions of the parents.

On the second day, the social worker met the psychiatrist at coffee and discussed further with him the parents' differences of opinion concerning placement of the boy. She said that the parents also felt the boy was aware of the possibility of placement and was anxious about it. The psychiatrist made a mental note to discuss placement with the boy. He then went on to report that he was impressed by the lessening of the boy's anxiety when he set firm limits as the psychologist had recommended. This information gave the social worker an important point to explore with the parents in order to discover what their own experiences were in regard to the boy's reaction to limits. The psychiatrist also mentioned that in his brief contacts with the parents when he called for the boy, the father wanted to impress upon him that the boy was "good" and could perform well. The social worker accepted these remarks as further indications of the father's insistence upon presenting the boy as normal and his wife as being at fault.

On the second day, the psychiatrist was also scheduled for a regular supervision hour; half of it was taken up with Harold's case, especially the evidence of brain damage. He discussed the limited information about this in the referring reports and his own impressions, but his supervisor suggested waiting until the neurologist had seen the boy before becoming too definite about such damage. (The psychiatrist had already shared the information known so far about the case with the neurologist, who was going to see the boy that afternoon.)

Later, toward the end of the second day, all the team members except the neurologist were in the general meeting room; present, too, was the senior psychologist who supervised the team psychologist. In a brief session, they tried to fit together their various observations. The social worker said:

> Harold's father doggedly insists on molding his son and labors under the belief that if he works hard enough and tries hard enough he can accomplish his goal. The reason for Harold's not living up to these expectations he then attributes to his wife, whom he blames for not being interested in the boy, not teaching him enough, and thus willfully depriving her husband of the gratification and satisfaction he needs from his son. Yet, Mrs. G. even plays baseball with Harold so he can become more acceptable to the children with whom he attempts to play. Mr. G. has revealed that unless he can help his son he will be a failure both as a father and as a man, and, therefore, the child simply has to be left in his care. The father's attitude has been "Harold can do it" because it is important for him that the child be adequate.

The psychologist commented that Harold kept saying "I can do it" and "Don't rush me." The boy felt under constant pressure to produce but would also say he could not. Nevertheless, he would try but resisted being pushed; he was anxious and had a constant need for reassurance from others. The boy asked not to be timed on the psychological tests, yet he had no real concept of time. At the age of nine years, six months, he failed some tasks at the five-year level; however, his understanding was quite good in some other areas at the eight-year-old level. The psychologist commented that he was becoming a little wary and wondered whether he would see the behavior the psychiatrist had mentioned, whether the boundaries would suddenly break and "the beautiful relationship would explode." So far, the boy had given in a little to him and he had given in a little to the boy; he would say, for example, "We'll do that again," and the boy would say, "No," but so far he had gone along. If, the psychologist said, he saw the boy was getting bored or the task was too rough for him, he modified his goal.

The psychiatrist again wondered whether the parents yet suspected brain damage, and the social worker replied they did not. She felt the parents were still very cautious and were afraid of criticism. She believed the father and mother would have a real tussle over the findings, and if there was brain damage, this might also present a serious problem for the mother because, during the pregnancy with this child, she had thought of having an abortion.

On the third day, the formal preconference (Chapter Eight) was held in the morning. The social worker briefly explained the child's relationship in the family (he had one sister nine years older) and summarized the background information about the child and parents and the reasons for referral, which we have reviewed. Among other things, she reported that the pregnancy, the delivery, and the child's very early development apparently were normal, with the exception of his club foot. The effects of this were probably considerable, however, as he was in a cast for fourteen months and was delayed in walking and talking. He entered the first grade at the usual time but the school thought he was not ready, so the parents obtained a private tutor. In later schooling, he was obviously promoted because of the effort he made. He could not play well with other children as he had poor coordination, and he usually sat by and watched them. Although the parents remained very guarded in the interviews, with questioning they would admit some of his difficulties; for instance, they said that they still had to cut his meat for him and tie his shoes. The social worker believed that some of the present difficulty arose because the mother tied the child to her in younger years and now was getting impatient and irritated with him. She went on to report that

an atmosphere of tension and dissatisfaction permeates this household and is threatening its structure and foundation. Probably they came to the clinic not only for Harold's sake but for their own— as individuals, rather than as a couple. Although these parents are undoubtedly caught in a dilemma because of the different advice of two professional people, their own mixed feelings toward their son and each other are also responsible for completely paralyzing them. They accuse each other for the child's deficiencies, which evoke feelings of inadequacy, guilt, and hostility in them; the child, of course, is caught in this tug-of-war and thus suffers almost the full brunt of their intense feelings. Mr. G. says his wife boycotts all his attempts to help Harold, and he speaks angrily of the frustration he experiences when faced with his wife's surface compliance but hidden resistance, which makes it impossible to "have things in the open." Mrs. G. does not display the overt hostility her husband shows; rather, she displays a meekness and a weariness that almost crush her to the ground. Unlike the tutor and family doctor, I don't feel this mother is near to being psychotic, but I do feel she is tired and worn out. The fact that we have not criticized her overtly has helped her to be more spontaneous and able to reveal very angry feelings toward Harold. My impression is that this mother's overprotectiveness is partly her way of counteracting the frightening hostility she feels toward the child. She sees him as a teary, whiny, demanding, clinging child, giving nothing and demanding everything. Mrs. G. seems lonely and lost in her family, having no one to turn to, always feeling she doesn't stand a chance. She says, for example, "My husband asks my opinion but overrides it. I might just as well have said nothing." There is apparently no real behavior problem with Harold, but he has other real difficulties in many areas and has fed upon the tension and strife in the home. It is impossible for the parents to tackle the problem with any unity, and this strife is also beginning to affect their daughter.

After team members asked a few questions about the social worker's impressions, the psychiatrist briefly described the boy and his interviews with him, supplying information on his intellectual deficits, his motor and perceptual difficulties, his anger and defiance when demands were thwarted, and his overall increased comfort in a structured situation. He stressed the boy's guardedness (he would give very little direct information about himself or his family), his anxiety about his level of performance, and his poor concept of himself. "He would frequently pretend we were twins (so we would start on an equal footing)," said the psychiatrist,

and we were supposed to be driving cars (he had to have the larger car). One of his favorite themes involved my driving on the wrong side of the road or doing some other careless thing that would result in my smashing into his car. He, of course, was driving faultlessly. He would insist that no one was hurt in the accident and would always excuse my negligence by remarking that anyone could have an accident. However, he is never really able to excuse himself for his own poor performance. For example, he once asked me to tie his shoestrings, explaining he couldn't quite learn how. He then pathetically asked me whether I had ever known another boy who couldn't tie his own shoes. Emotionally, his prevailing mood is one of anxious uncertainty about what will be asked of him and his ability to comply. At one point, he became frustrated when he was unable to hit the punching bag on the rebound. His first reaction was to say that it didn't work well, and then to add it was no fun anyway. In playing horseshoes, he might explain, "Mine are closer to the stake than yours, aren't they? I did better than you," even though his horseshoes might be three feet farther away than mine. I don't feel he actually believed this, but I suspect he is accustomed to receiving parental affirmation of his superiority even when this is by no means the case.

The neurologist reported that the child was quite tense and fearful during his examination but offered no major resistance to it. His initial diagnosis was encephalopathy, diffuse and congenital, caused by unknown factors, and manifested by retarded mental and motor development. There were mild, nonspecific deficits in motor coordination, and the left foot was smaller than the right, with a suggestive bilateral peroneal muscle weakness. The neurologist did not feel that the boy's club foot had much to do with his coordination difficulties, which, he believed, were related more to his brain condition. Laboratory studies, however, had not yet been completed.

The psychologist next reported a picture quite similar to that of the examining psychiatrist. The results of the tests so far suggested that Harold was intellectually quite limited, particularly in the perceptual-motor area, where his performance strongly suggested organic brain impairment. So far, his abilities ranged from the five- to the nine-year level. Even measured by the five-year level, he had difficulty in folding a piece of paper into a triangle. He was unable to copy from memory a bead-chain design requiring the simple alternation of square and round forms. He barely was able to draw a square (five-year level)', and completely unable to draw a diamond (seven-year level)'. On the Bender-Gestalt, his figures were not only extremely primitive, but in two drawings, he broke up the Gestalt so that his copies were completely fragmented and disorganized, suggesting organic impairment rather than simple retardation.

Another aspect suggesting organic impairment was his rigidity and inability to shift flexibly from one area to another. Thus, in attempting to put together a puzzle normally passed at the three-year level, he was unable to continue because he had one of the pieces upside down. It was not until the examiner asked him to close his eyes and turned the piece around for him that he was able to break the mental set and put the piece in place. Many of his responses had a perseverative, or repetitive, quality and he had a markedly concrete orientation to the world. The psychologist also reported that the boy's behavior was frequently quite infantile; he reacted with immediate anger when demands were not met, was whiny, and refused to continue the task at hand. He was restless, distractible, and easily fatigued.

The team then had a general discussion and considered such questions as what reaction members might expect from the parents as they began to share their findings with them. They also considered the possibilities for the boy's future development; for example, they did not rule out the possibility that he might eventually be able to learn a simple trade. They also made tentative recommendations on the case and agreed that the parents should place less stress on academic performance and that demands on the child should be geared more to his ability. Emphasis was also laid on the need for a more structured environment for him and continued attention to the parents' problems as they affected him. Such factors as the mother's menopausal depression were also considered.

From this preconference the social worker now knew that her next tasks were to begin to share the findings directly with the parents and help them learn about their son's serious organic impairment, to handle the emotional impact of this, and to begin to discuss with them the effect that the implications of these findings should have on their attitudes toward the boy, their attitudes toward themselves, and their attitudes toward each other. The father, for example, could no longer justifiably push the boy so hard or feel that it was a reflection on him if the boy did not become normal.

Neither would he be able to use the boy so directly as a weapon against the mother. The social worker's third task was to explore tentatively what the findings meant in relation to treatment recommendations. These might include placing less pressure on the boy to perform, providing a firmer environmental structure for him, and probably not separating him from the home—at least not until he was given a chance to respond to what would hopefully be a shift in the parents' attitudes and management of him.

Each of the team members in this preconference received validation from the others of their findings. The neurologist had still to obtain the laboratory studies, the psychologist had yet to complete the test battery he had selected to use with the boy, and the psychiatrist had to continue his diagnostic and therapeutic endeavors in order to obtain a rounded picture of the child and help him as much as possible (that is, help him with feelings about himself and his general problems and with his concerns about the examination and then prepare him for the termination of this process). The team psychiatrist also had to be available to the social worker to help with the sharing and interpretation of the findings to the parents. Of course, the social worker had already laid the groundwork for this effort in previous interviews by questioning the parents about Harold's performance difficulties. These questions were based on the information she had obtained early in the process from the psychiatrist and psychologist.

Later, on the third day, the psychologist met with the psychiatrist and reported that in an unstructured situation, such as with the Rorschach which he had just given Harold, the boy became very anxious and difficult to manage—behaving, in fact, much as he did when the psychiatrist first saw him. Also on this day, the social worker discussed the case with her supervisor. The worker felt that the mother was disappointed because the team was not recommending a separation at this time. On the other hand, the father in his interview after the preconference talked of temporary separation from the boy and felt that his wife needed a rest. He seemed to be less critical of his wife and much more positive toward the clinic. The social worker felt this change may have occurred because of the information she had begun to share with him about the actual condition of the boy—his brain damage and inherent limitations. In response, the social work supervisor discussed with the team social worker how to proceed in the directions emerging from the preconference.

On the fourth day, the social worker saw the psychiatrist and mentioned to him the parents' request that he be the one to discuss the recommendations with Harold. She felt they wanted the psychiatrist to do their job, but, at the same time, she also felt that there was some kind of new communication between the parents, and with the boy, too. For instance, for the first time they were observed talking to each other while waiting for their appointments. She also reported the change she felt in Mr. G.; he was less defensive and more accepting of the findings. His wife was stunned by the findings, but in a gruff way he had tried to reassure her. The social worker felt that with a noncritical attitude—neither oversupporting or otherwise—she would be able to help them both to accept the situation and to begin to plan for it. The psychiatrist also shared with the social worker the information that the psychologist had given him about the child's becoming more disturbed during the Rorschach examination, along with the psychologist's ideas on the possible implications.

Later on this day, the team psychologist briefly talked over his findings and final report with the supervising psychologist. The team psychologist also sought out the team social worker and psychiatrist, reading to them the CAT (Children's Apperception Test) responses of the child, which revealed some of the boy's attitudes toward his parents; for example, the boy saw the parent figures in many of the pictures as scolding and angry. The psychiatrist, in turn, described the boy's aggressive behavior with some of the toys that seemed to represent the members of his family; he kicked and hit, for example, the large air-filled "Bobo" figure.

By putting together this information from each discipline, the team members were able to come to some conclusions about how much the parents' behavior actually corresponded with their son's perceptions. The social work process and the interaction among the family members helped the team learn that the parents actually pushed the boy to perform beyond his capabilities. Some-

times they were impatient with him or swung to the other extreme
of being overindulgent. Harold's free play with the psychiatrist and
the results from the psychologist's projective tests revealed how
much the boy's inner attitudes colored what he perceived. This revelation furnished important clues for determining whether external,
environmental, and parental changes might be all that the boy
needed to help him or whether psychotherapy was also necessary for
altering his strongly internalized attitudes.

On the fifth day of the study, a final conference was held.
Since the team had discussed the reasons for referral, the referring
reports, relevant family background information, the life history of
the child, and the present situation in the preconference, they dealt
with them only very briefly here. Then, the social worker concentrated on describing her further process with the parents. She
pointed out the marked changes in the father after she had begun
to share the findings with him. (What she was forgetting, of course,
was that the movement toward change had actually begun in her
very first session with the parents and was shaped and influenced
by the tone and atmosphere she had set.) "The father actually related warmly to me," the social worker said,

> almost releasing his clenched fists, so to speak. Now he saw his son
> as a demanding and difficult child who was wearing out both his
> wife and himself, and he even hinted that they needed a rest from
> the boy to collect themselves and face the "newly found truths."
> Moreover, the process had helped the father to be less threatened
> by the findings; now he could really look at them, accept them,
> and, in a way, hear them for the first time, so that in a sense they
> were new to him. Actually he must have been aware of much of
> the truth all along—knowing but not knowing, as it were. But
> even though he now accepted the findings, he still spoke of the
> great shock he had experienced from realizing his son's slowness
> and that tutoring would not bridge the gap scholastically. He also
> said that he understood his wife's feeling of helplessness, which
> he had previously always attacked as laziness or indifference. During
> the last few days, both Mr. and Mrs. G. have been able to talk to
> each other about Harold's difficulties and recognize their own as
> well as the child's problems without feeling they are failures.

The social worker added that the parents' ability to take hold of the casework contacts made her feel they could benefit from further clinical work in their attempts to live with the fact that their child was slow. She also believed that they would benefit from securing help for themselves.

After a few questions and a brief discussion, the psychiatrist gave his report, adding new developments. For example, he reported the boy's great concern with anything that was broken. "He asked with real feeling," he said, "how the teddy bear had lost an eye, and he showed the same concern over a broken leg on one of the dolls and about a car door that wouldn't open." He also commented on the boy's almost complete lack of awareness of sexual differences. "He informed me that men are different from women because their hair is different, and he once remarked, 'Let's pretend we're married.' Further questioning revealed that he thought this entirely possible and saw no reason why men shouldn't marry each other and have children." On the other hand, the psychiatrist observed that the boy gave indirect evidence of being more aware of family disturbances and parental conflict than he would openly express. But he still looked to his parents, particularly his mother, for much protection and support. He seemed to rely less on his father and to be more frightened of him.

The psychologist reported on Harold's increased tension during the projective tests, the easy regression to infantile behavior, and the difficulty he had with control. "On the fourth day, his obdurate resistance, imperiousness, impatience, and need to structure the situation according to his wishes become clear—characteristics only hinted at previously. It was difficult, in fact, for me to be able to control his behavior sufficiently to obtain the necessary material. His responses on the Rorschach were of poor quality, being primitive and perseverative. His tension tolerance was extremely low, and in a situation where no boundaries existed he regressed to such a primitive level of functioning that his aggressive impulses were almost uncontrolled. Even when limits were rather rigidly set, he became impatient very easily, like a much younger child." The psychologist then went on to say that his stories on the CAT suggested that he felt he was punished for his ineptness and, apparently, often spanked because of it. They also suggested that he felt his parents were dissatisfied with him. A number of them dealt with the same theme: A child falls into the lake, comes home wet and dirty, and gets spanked by his father or mother. He expressed considerable aggression toward both parents: "I bite when I get mad," he said. "When I get so mad, I want to hurt someone—Daddy or someone." It was also necessary for him to deny these aggressive feelings which he blurted out. Further, his stories suggested his confusion and uncertainty about his parents' dependability and his feelings about which of them was really on his side. Oedipal conflict was also hinted at in the story he told about "a tiger who came to the king and threw the king out and took his chair." In regard to his overall performance, he functioned at a borderline to dull-normal level.

Next, the neurologist reported that the EEG and skull X-rays were negative; team members, however, agreed that the clinical findings from the other disciplines, as well as neurology, had shown evidence of organic factors in the boy's difficulties. They then discussed how disturbed the boy was. The psychologist noted that as Harold became more secure, his demands became more insistent even in structured situations. The team felt that the boy was used to having exorbitant demands made on him and that if the demands could be decreased possibly he could relax his own demands. Until now, apparently related to his own concerns about adequacy, the father's acceptance of the child was very much tied up with what Harold could do. If the parents could get help with these and other problems, the team believed the total family situation might be considerably improved. The social worker had discussed such help with the parents and they recognized a need for it after she had shown them how they were using the boy in their struggles with each other. Members felt that the boy would need psychotherapy along with whatever help he would get from environmental changes such as the parents putting less pressure on the boy to perform beyond his capacities.

Thus, the final conference produced new information, with team members reporting the following:

1. Laboratory studies were normal, but there was clinical evidence of brain damage.

2. The boy's conscious and less conscious attitudes toward his parents and others had become clearer.

3. The boy responded somewhat differently to the psychologist than he had to the psychiatrist, even when the latter provided a structured situation. The boy was probably less healthy than was supposed at the time of the preconference.

4. The parents showed significant shifts in attitudes.

At this final conference, team members also arrived at these final diagnostic conclusions:

1. The child was both brain-damaged and intellectually retarded, with unevenness in the degree of damage and retardation in different areas.

2. The degree of internal emotional disturbance associated with the boy's brain damage and retardation was impossible to assess satisfactorily, because concomitant external factors were creating additional stress and anxiety for him at the present time.

3. The disturbance between the parents (the nature of which was difficult to clarify entirely) was one factor preventing them from viewing and treating the child realistically and, therefore, was causing him unnecessary anxiety.

From these diagnostic considerations the team members made these final recommendations:

1. The child should have a special educational program geared to his individual needs in school, but separation from the family did not appear to be indicated at this time, either from the child's or from the parents' point of view. (If the father could take the pressure off his wife and son, Mrs. G. might feel less need to place her son in a special home, and the son might create fewer problems.)

2. Psychotherapy for the boy was indicated.

3. The parents should obtain casework help for themselves in working out their difficulties with each other, so they could stop using the boy in their personal struggle.

In the postconference interview with the parents, the psychiatrist and the social worker did not have to share many new findings with Mr. and Mrs. G. since they had already discussed this information with them following the preconference. During the conversation the father stated that he had been laboring under the false assumption that his wife could do something for Harold, but he recognized now that the child had certain limitations. The mother immediately commented that she had been overprotective of Harold but had always felt pushed to be so because of his handicap.

Many questions now came up about what the boy would be capable of doing. The psychiatrist and the social worker outlined his capabilities for the parents, stressing that they should return to their local guidance center and explore some of these problems still further as they arose. The psychiatrist and the social worker agreed with both parents that the child could be quite difficult at times, and although he was also at times friendly and pleasant, his constant demands and needs could be very draining. Recognition of this situation by the psychiatrist and the social worker helped the parents to relax and to feel more comfortable about their dissatisfaction and irritation with him. The parents then got into some disagreement about whether or not Harold should be made to eat specific foods, and the social worker used their argument as an indication of why they needed further help to answer the many comparable questions that would arise once they were home. These disagreements were also the basis for again pointing out the usefulness of considering the possibility of securing help with their own problems with each other.

Before the parents left, they both stated that they felt they had gained a great deal from their stay. They felt much more comfortable now that they had a better understanding of what to expect of the boy and knew which way to turn. Some of their fear of being failures because the child was unable to live up to their expectations had diminished markedly. They expressed again the tremendous shock this recognition had been to them, but they also felt ready to work with it. They were pleased that we would be communicating with the guidance center they had previously contacted about our findings, and they said that they were planning to return there. A follow-up report confirmed that they had contacted the agency and were working out arrangements for help.

How had the team been able to work successfully with this

family, when previous attempts had apparently failed? First of all, it is impossible to assess the extent of insight for which previous helpers were responsible. Even when the parents could not completely face the situation, each previous contact probably brought them a little closer to being ready to deal with the psychological truth. Of course, time itself must absorb the depressing and deeply injurious blow that parents of a damaged child feel. The time factor is extremely important and became active the moment Mr. and Mrs. G. first sought guidance with their child.

In regard to the help that the clinic gave, "success" was not accomplished so quickly or so simply as it might appear; as previously stressed, it is impossible to convey the intensive process undertaken with this family, particularly in the interviews that the social worker had with the parents. No doubt, the comprehensiveness of the examination was also a significant factor in helping the father deal more realistically with what he was really aware of all along, that the child was inherently handicapped and was not being held back primarily by maternal overprotection or rejection. Mr. G.'s having to live with the boy for twenty-four hours a day for five days may have forced him to an increased awareness of his son's actual handicaps and the draining effect they had upon those around him. The noncritical, supporting role of the team members was also extremely important. It enabled this insecure father to accept the idea of a child with limited abilities and not to experience this problem as a sign of personal failure. Very significant, too, was the fact that Mr. and Mrs. G. had enough strength to make use of this kind of help when it was offered them.

INDIVIDUAL CONTRIBUTIONS

In this case illustration, we see a reasonably effective team operation, although, as stated at the beginning, the team members were relatively inexperienced and at times were anxious about what they could accomplish. But from the help and support they were able to derive from each other, as well as from their supervisors and conference leaders, they were able to offer real assistance to a confused and mutually defeating family. The advantages of approaching the problem through an interdisciplinary effort can be further highlighted by considering the individual contributions of the team members.

In this case, it was clearly necessary to have a neurologist evaluate the possibility of possible brain damage. Although the psychiatrist and the psychologist contributed to this area too, an adequate study demanded neurological and laboratory tests to give a more complete picture of the problem. A neurological evaluation is not something that can be satisfactorily carried out by the psychiatrist, even though he is a medical person, unless he also happens to be particularly trained and experienced in doing neurological examinations of children, and most psychiatrists are not. Had a neurological study been done before the family considered the clinic, it might have helped prevent the conflict that arose between the two early examiners—the psychologist and the tutor. As mentioned before, the latter had originally suspected brain damage, but apparently because of a change in some of the boy's symptoms, he had decided that more functional difficulties stemming from the mother-child interaction were responsible for the boy's behavior. Nor had the report from the boy's family physician to the clinic made mention of possible brain damage.

A full understanding of the case could not have been achieved, either, without the significant contributions of the child psychologist, who extensively assessed the child's various levels of functioning under different kinds of stimulus and demand. He was able to give a fuller, more precise, and more differentiated picture of some of the child's psychological assets and liabilities than either the neurologist or psychiatrist could provide with their techniques. Such a differential assessment is of the greatest importance in future planning for the child, since it provides an estimate of the level at which he can work, evaluates the areas in which he can be expected to do better, and considers which areas should be less emphasized. Again, perhaps part of the difficulty in the past with this case arose because the tutor obtained, from the limited test battery he administered, a considerably higher score than was found by the psychologist who had previously tested the boy. As a result, the tutor underplayed the boy's inherent limitations. Finality cannot be attributed to the IQ, because some variation is known to exist in the results from time to time, from test to test, and from examiner to examiner—especially with disturbed children and children with unbalanced capacities. We could rely on test results of the team psychologist because (1) he administered a wider range of tests from which to draw his conclusions than had ever been given to the boy before and (2) test findings correlated closely with the clinical impressions of the psychiatrist and the neurologist.

In addition to the valuable findings added by the psychologist concerning specific effects of brain damage and areas of intellectual retardation, he also made other important contributions. For example, he was able to contribute to further understanding of how the child felt both about himself and others from his responses on the CAT. These responses were particularly helpful because Harold resisted the psychiatrist's direct exploration of such topics and only infrequently acted out such themes with the family dolls, unlike many other children. Another type of useful information the psychologist provided was the boy's initial response to structure, along with the discovery that even with set limits he would rather quickly become difficult to manage if pressed to perform or asked to deal with such anxiety-arousing material as the Rorschach.

The staff psychiatrist also served several necessary functions. First, he took the overall medical responsibility for the complete case and for the child's physical assessment, which, along with the more specific neurological studies, is vital to the process. He served an important function as well in assisting the social worker in the discussion of the medical aspects of the case with the parents. He also obtained, insofar as possible, a history directly from the child. There are obvious advantages to having this story, in addition to that obtained from the parents. Moreover, the psychiatrist obtained useful information from the free-play situation in his office and from his relationship with the boy—information that both supplemented and confirmed the material acquired by the neurologist, the psychologist, and the social worker.

In his therapeutic function with the boy (Meyers, 1956; Modlin, Gardner, and Faris, 1958), the psychiatrist was able to help him cope with his doubts about himself, his anger toward his parents and the insecurity he experienced with them, and his misunderstanding and apprehensions about the clinic examinations; he also prepared him for terminating his new relationships at the clinic.

As part of her contribution to the case, the social worker obtained information about the family background, the child's development and his reactions to his sister, peers, school, and other social situations. She obtained a picture of the child as each parent viewed him and gained an impression of each parent and their interactions with each other and with their child. In addition to presenting to the team an incisive glimpse of the family—a glimpse that conveyed the intensity of their struggle within themselves and with each other and their attitudes toward the study—she furnished members such realities of the family situation as the nature of the community in which they lived, the availability of local resources, and their financial situation.

In addition, the social worker dealt empathically with the parents' conscious and unconscious resistance to the helping process and brought out and strengthened their desire to get help. We saw, for example, how she assisted the mother by providing realistic information about Harold's limitations, which helped her to see she was not the reason for his lack of progress. Similarly, the social worker assisted the father by helping him to see that if the child's performance was inadequate this was not a reflection on either his wife or himself. She assisted them both in their relationship to each other by helping them realize what they were doing to each other, to question their motivations, and to recognize that the way they were doing it (through the child) was destructive to all of them. She was able to help them change, to modify the way they were abusing each other, so they at least could become more communicative and understanding with each other, and could work with some unity on both the child's problems and theirs.

From the above discussion, we see the many areas that must be cooperatively explored in order to achieve a comprehensive understanding of the child and his family, and to use this understanding with the family effectively. A wide range of special skills and techniques are required along with adequate time and opportunity in which to use and integrate them—especially for cases with complex difficulties. This wide range of potentialities inherent in the team makes possible flexible and unified services to meet individual case needs.

When special examinations and reports must be independently obtained from various specialists in different agencies, the result is often that the family is seen sectionally and no true synthesis is achieved. In our case example, several people had previously seen the family; each was aware of the other's reports, but in no way were these reports integrated. The parents were also aware of the separate reports, and this knowledge only added to their separate ways of viewing the problem. Generally, the different disciplines can function best when they take into account each other's findings *during* the time that their own process is being conducted. For example, in this case we saw how important it was for the social worker to have data that gave a clear view of the boy's actual capacities—data that she could use early in her process with the parents. Similarly, information supplied by the social worker about how the parents felt and dealt with the boy contributed to the psychiatrist's understanding. Thus, when the team members work together in an integrating process, each member of the interdisciplinary team can maximize his understanding and help to the family throughout the process.

Moreover, when a number of team members with various backgrounds and training are working together, there is a greater opportunity to counteract blind spots and biases (Caudill, 1958; Dittes and Kelley, 1956). Countertransference feelings and reactions are an inevitable part of the process, but what is not inevitable is that they go unrecognized and interfere with constructive work. Functioning in a group requires an exposure of each person's work to the view of the other members, which places checks and balances upon it. Sometimes the charge is made that the team separates the parents from the child, and, to some extent, probably the use of such techniques as joint interviews and family therapy has arisen out of an attempt to prevent this separation. In a well-integrated team, however, taking sides or seeing the family members too much apart from each other does not occur. It is probably more likely to occur when one individual works alone with the family, without the corrections that group scrutiny provides. As mentioned in the case of Harold and the parents, the previous examiners had been "split" in their opinions, just as the parents were. Our team members did not allow the family to force them to take sides, because they did not view their processes separately. In the beginning of any process, each team member is somewhat preoccupied with his own examination, but he soon feels the need for the impressions of the others. Then, the members work through their varied experiences—similar and conflicting—and move toward an integration of all the contributions. Each member of the family is similarly helped to shift his viewpoint and come to a consensus with the other family members. In other words, the team provides the family with an identification group that is not split by conflict and this, in turn, helps the family members to resolve their conflicts and become reunited.

We do not mean to imply that differences never occur in the findings among the team members. In fact, differences may become so clear that the team will also discuss them with the family. Team members may show that fact A carries such a weight and that fact B also carries such a weight that they are unable to reconcile them. That both A and B can be observed shows how multifactored the problem is and how multifactored the solution may need to be. Often, when a family sees that the team respects differences they are encouraged to respect their own differences.

Our case has also illustrated the contribution of the team experiences to training. Teaching and learning go hand in hand in every case, whether formally or informally, from the regular performance of team functions. The knowledge and insight each individual derives from working with other disciplines and seeing a problem from other points of view, as well as from his own, enrich his experience. The requirement to function out in the open may make for more careful work and also insures that the work of inexperienced members, who may receive assistance from more senior team members, will come up to a sufficiently high caliber. Although

the presence of trainees will to some extent slow down and hamper
the other team members, this is a price that has to be paid in
training, no matter how it is done.

Another aspect of teamwork—a subtle one—concerns mo-
rale and work satisfaction. Despite some anxieties connected with
working in a group, most people find teamwork is usually stim-
ulating and rewarding. The educational gains, the satisfaction
from shared effort, and the security resulting from carrying out a
comprehensive instead of a single study make it a good way of
working in many instances. A team can also often tolerate the
stresses and strains involved in psychiatric diagnostic work with
children better than the inexperienced individual working alone.
When the full impact of a problem has to be borne by one individual he may feel too burdened to deal with it effectively, but
shared with the team, it may be reduced to a manageable size.

In summary, we have presented a brief illustration of the
functioning of an interdisciplinary diagnostic team. The usefulness
of this approach is only fully realized in a well-functioning team,
however. When problems of one sort or another interfere in its
smooth operations, its effectiveness will be reduced. We will now
turn to a consideration of such problems.

TEAM MISFUNCTION

Before considering some of the problems that can arise in
teamwork, we would like to emphasize that difficulties of some kind
are bound to occur in any type of group collaboration, whether
it is a family, a faculty department, or a research team. Many of
these problems are by no means related only to the psychiatric
diagnostic team. Professional people are not superhuman. They are
as subject as anyone else to ups and downs, good days and bad
days, and distracting personal problems. With them, as in any
group, there may be angry feelings, competitive struggles, resent-
ments, efforts of one person to dominate another, and differences
in judgment and in willingness to take the lead or share responsibility. But because of the nature of the psychiatric team's work—
with its frequent emotional stresses and pressures, which can
seriously affect the family—it is more vital for team members to

deal effectively with these problems than it is for some other professional team groups. Teamwork in certain ways requires even more flexibility and maturity than psychiatric work done alone. When the psychiatric professional works by himself, his ups and downs and lapses of attention are not observable to anyone but himself (or, unfortunately, sometimes to his patients), and he may even rationalize the difficulties sufficiently to be unaware of them. However, in teamwork, these temporary or recurrent difficulties are not only visible to the other members but sometimes affect the group effort as a whole. However, with reasonably good rapport, team members can usually handle minor problems, as sufficient willingness to take turns in sharing the burden prevails then and makes up for whatever weak spots exist at a given time.

Most of the problems of interdisciplinary team functioning are not inherent in the process itself. A number of other factors, including problems within the individual and the larger setting in which the team works, may be involved. The importance of the influence of the society within which the psychiatric team works has become well recognized (Caudill, 1958). Individually and as a team, members are sensitive to factors beyond what is going on in their own group. If they feel that other demands are at variance with their own, they may have trouble (Thelen, 1956). Problems may arise in connection with status, disagreement over roles, or in having to carry out several roles, some of which may conflict. When an individual is also a member of another group which is pressed by conflict, or when the decision of one group depends on that of another, cross-pressures may ensue. For example, disagreement between the staff of the inpatient service and the staff of the diagnostic service over the kinds of children to be admitted for treatment may hamper the diagnostic team.

Difficulties may also carry over from previous interactions or may result from team members' work on other cases or even from other areas outside the diagnostic service. For example, residual feelings about a social worker's previous failure to share in an unrelated treatment situation may persist and distort the reaction of the psychiatrist working with him on a diagnostic case. Individual problems and idiosyncrasies may also interfere in group functioning. For instance, a psychologist may repeatedly spend more time than scheduled with a patient, "forgetting" others had also scheduled appointments and were kept waiting. (Not infrequently, the individual may project his own problems onto the group, and, similarly, the group may project its difficulties onto an individual, or onto some other situation outside the group.)

New members of a team may also contribute a variety of difficulties to the group (Modlin and Faris, 1956), including those relating to his inexperience in the field and those that arise inevitably just because he is a newcomer, regardless of his training and experience (Ziller and Behringer, 1960). When any individual joins a group, several steps occur. First, he will attempt to find his place, where he fits in, what will be expected of him, and what he can expect of the group. At the same time, the group members will be examining him in a similar light. During this early period, certain conflicts may arise over the differences between the new individual's wishes and expectations and those of the group. Gradually, attempts will be made to resolve some of the conflicts emerging from these differences. Eventually, more productive work will be done as these difficulties are ironed out.

There is naturally a difference in the ease with which people adapt themselves when entering a new group as well as a difference in how groups accept new members (Ziller and Belringer, 1961); some individuals are able to be flexible and adjust quickly, others need more time. Initially, a new member may be somewhat self-centered, his attention focused more on his own need for orientation than on the needs of the team. Later, when he has learned the ropes, he has more energy to invest in the work of the team, because he is spending less time on his own problems. Some inexperienced new members may lack appreciation for the value of working with a team. They may even feel that the team gets in the way of their working more directly with the family and thus be unwilling to invest much effort on the group. Or, more likely, they may intellectually accept the team concept without having a genuine feeling for it. Understanding and belief in its value come only from experiencing the team method in successful work.

Some of the new member's problems arise from the "family"

structure of the team, with its older and younger members and its hierarchies of authority and responsibility. Even in the most mature and well-functioning team, disguised family feelings may be present without ordinarily interfering. A new member is an unknown quantity, and the less secure members may see him as a threat or have unrealistic expectations for him; then, resentment and distrust may grow and be expressed openly or subtly when he does not reach these expectations. Sometimes, it is safer to criticize a junior member than someone more senior; thus, anger felt toward the latter may be displaced to the former.

Another occasional problem is rooted in the feelings of team members toward their peers; these may be expressed in interruptions or arguments, which confuse the thinking of the group. A team member may even displace child-parent conflicts, by reacting to a team leader or supervisor as he might to a parent with whom he must passively comply, compete for, or aggressively oppose. There may also be an overeagerness to please and to accept the views of the senior members, or the junior members may present what they believe the leaders will want to hear, regardless of whether this is what they actually believe themselves.

The older members are responsible for helping the new members and increasing their security; however, if the older members themselves have unresolved conflicts, they may in one way or another extract a "payment" from the new member for letting him into the "club." For example, they may give the new members the "dirty work" to do, such as writing up the meetings, or they may keep the junior members or new members in less important roles than they should be playing.

When a member is not only new to a team but also inexperienced, further complications are naturally added. However, the deficiency of the inexperienced new member is partly compensated for by the more senior team members and by supervision. When even with this help the inexperienced member for one reason or another cannot fulfill his expected role, major problems will arise. These problems may be especially difficult for the junior psychiatrist, who in many settings is traditionally made the team leader, even though he is new and inexperienced and even though members of other disciplines are more experienced and better qualified to lead. Inevitably, then, strain arises.

The problem of unjustified conformity to someone else's viewpoint or to the group's opinion is an important one in team-work, because then the full advantages of a team cannot be realized (Dittes and Kelley, 1956; Tuddenham, 1958). The individual who is confident of himself and of his position with his associates will feel free to present evidence differing from the other members or to change his understanding; when this confidence is present, the tendency to apply the usual pressures against deviation would probably be diminished.

A new member may try to deal with insecurity in other ways than by an inhibited, unsure approach. For example, a new and relatively inexperienced member may present a facade of dogmatic certainty. He may search for "key words" and report "sudden insights," about which the more experienced team members may become suspicious, feeling that many of his formulations are not based on enough evidence and are too theoretical to be of any practical value. Here, the new member is handling his anxiety by intellectualizing and by working too independently of the team. Of course, new members can usually sense whether the others consider them to be doing well or not. The opinions of peers and leaders are, of course, extremely important, and disapproval from them may be reacted to and defended against in various ways (Zander, Stotland, and Wolfe, 1960). One way the low-status member has of dealing with the group's not accepting him is to devaluate the group; another way, and an opposite reaction, is to devaluate oneself.

Another aspect we would like to consider is the problem of new members being unduly influenced by the family they are evaluating. This can, of course, occur to experienced workers, too, and involves the question of countertransference which cannot be considered in detail here. (It is also necessary to keep in mind the differences between countertransference reactions and the many other ways a worker can react to a family and make use of them in unhealthful ways. For example, a worker may try to use his process with the family to bolster his own self-esteem by winning the team's praise for his "success"; his need to succeed thus interferes with his objective approach to the family. Or he may use his process with the family as a weapon against other members of the team—that is, to assert his authority or to "show up" another's process as being inferior to his own. These reactions are not countertransference problems with the real family; they are, if anything, more like countertransference problems within the team "family.")

Certain difficulties or patterns in the family can so influence team members that they are prevented from understanding or helping the family to the fullest extent possible (Brodey and Hayden, 1957). As an example, we may use a situation in which the prognosis is poor or in which no treatment resources are available. In our culture—a culture that is essentially optimistic and expects everything to turn out well, *especially* for our children—the impact of the seriously emotionally disturbed child and his parents on the team members can be very great. This problem may be particularly hard for younger members when they have difficulty in accepting the limitations of help that can be given. They may have trouble in giving up their unrealistic hopes and fantasies about what they can accomplish, or they may have a problem in facing the limitations of the field itself (Rettig, Jacobson, and Pasamanick, 1958).

The consensus of the team can help in whatever irrational doubts and guilt a team member may feel about a case. Other members may support him by stressing that everyone has done his best under the circumstances. Generally, difficult situations are better tolerated by the group than by the individual (Lichtenberg, 1957). Some members react differently to different problems and can deal with one aspect better than another; thus some can be supporting in one case and fail to be in another. In any event, the older and more experienced individuals can be of support to the junior and less experienced team members, who are most subject to unrealistic optimism or pessimism, or to anger or guilt. These reactions must be recognized and dealt with before the team can move ahead. While much can be said for youthful optimism, certain realities must be faced. It would be a mistake to require a family to make unrealistic sacrifices to support treatment from which no hope of success is possible.

Another difficulty arises when a parent arouses hostility in a team member. For instance, in one case, which we shall refer to as the *M. case,* a psychiatric resident not even working directly with the family developed considerable hostility toward the child's mother. During the preconference he commented, "It would be hard to work with this woman without becoming angry." The chairman replied that one had to free oneself of anger to work with her, and the social work supervisor pointed out that the mother was very frightened. A little later, the resident commented, "Her attitude is really a destructive one"; and when the psychologist began playing a recording of the boy's peculiar voice, he burst out with much feeling, "You ought to tell the mother she doesn't have to drive this boy insane. He's already organically damaged."

In this instance, the trainee had lost his objectivity under the pressure of anxiety at hearing the child's strange voice and had angrily sided with the child against the mother. Such an attitude is frequently observed in less experienced workers who overlook the multiplicity of causal factors. They simply blame the mother and father for the child's difficulties, without being sufficiently aware of the parents' own problems or without fully comprehending the struggle they are having with the child; they are not yet sensitized to the complicated interaction that goes on between the parents and child to create a family problem. However, the new worker may, instead, be receptive to the parents to the exclusion of the child. Of course, many variations and combinations are possible (Bornstein, 1948). Such attitudes prevent both seeing the case in its totality and finding the necessary solutions for the total problem. Those who work with children and, thus, are especially prone to overidentification must learn not to become so involved that they are too angry, too depressed, or too sympathetic to give objective help. There is also the opposite danger of becoming overly callous and indifferent as a defense against the pain and suffering that even training and experience cannot relieve. The checks and balances inherent in functioning as a team aid in minimizing these over- or underreactions to the family or to some of its members.

So far, we have concentrated on problems arising with individual team members—particularly new and inexperienced ones; this picture is out of focus because such difficulties also exert a greater or lesser effect on the other team members and on the group as a whole. In any team, collectively and individually, many things are going on besides the actual job at hand. An overt and a covert process are always present (Thelen, 1956). The overt process is that of trying to understand and help the family; the covert process is made up of many other goals, struggles, reactions, and wishes that are related to needs of the individual members and of the group, rather than to the needs of the family. Competition with a co-worker, rebellion against the leader's authority, the wish to impress a supervisor, resentment of a colleague—these feelings and others like them are "extracurricular," covert issues present in every process (LeBarre, 1960; Whitman, 1956). Some of these reactions all the team members consciously feel, some only certain members experience and, on occasion, subtle factors that prevent full concentration on the task at hand escape everyone's conscious awareness. At times, conflicts which openly involve some members of the team more than others may be secretly supported and nourished by those members who, without risking actual involvement, indirectly find the tension gratifying.

The team's goal must be to help the family, but when the unconscious goal is to struggle with inner team conflicts, the focus, as a consequence, is too internalized; the covert process becomes too dominant and the work with the family suffers. Failure results, then, when the team uses the case process to meet its own needs rather than for the diagnosis and treatment of the family. A certain degree of team introspection is necessary for good team function, but too much involvement or conflict with each other, regardless of the reason, will make the total process suffer.

An example of this type of problem arose in the T. case, in which the psychiatrist became too involved in the psychologist's difficulties. At a certain stage the psychology trainee—possibly from anxiety about adequately fulfilling his role—told the psychiatric trainee that he was having difficulty getting the child's responses on the Rorschach. In his next session with the child, the psychiatric trainee spent his time making inkblots on paper and inquiring about what the girl saw. Not surprisingly, this experiment backfired and the child refused to come in for her next session with the psychiatrist. She did return, however, to see the psychologist. In this case, the psychiatric trainee either felt too great a need to help the psychology trainee or—and more likely—he unconsciously wanted to show the psychologist that he (or psychiatry) could do a better job.

Of course, the family being studied may also come with the overt goal of getting help but still may have extracurricular covert purposes—again, individually and as a group—that both interact and interfere with this goal. These covert purposes, such as to prove that one parent is right and the other is wrong or that the child is not sick, may seriously affect or nullify the team's efforts to help.

Another important aspect of team functioning is the willingness on the part of the members to change. While a certain amount of stability and structure is necessary, too much rigidity prevents growth. The team may settle down to working in a certain way even though it is not the best way, or they may agree simply because it is easier or more comfortable to agree than to disagree (Eiduson, 1966). Team agreement and self-satisfaction, then, may not always be indicative of good work. Unspoken patterns of group culture sometimes determine the interactions and communications in the team to an excessive degree, whereas the major determinant should be what is needed in a particular case to facilitate understanding, so that the parents and child can be helped. Thus, to reach this goal, some of the ordinary patterns that characterize the relationship of members may have to be altered; if, however, these patterns are too fixed in hierarchies or too determined by personal alliances or rivalries, such a change cannot occur.

Among the many other important factors in team functioning that we might discuss are such questions as group size and composition and the requirements necessary for maximum creativity (Thelen, 1956). However, we will turn our attention instead to three specific areas that are of great significance in the functioning of the interdisciplinary diagnostic team. These include the differentiation and integration of team member's roles, leadership, and communication.

Confusion of Roles

We have previously referred to dilemmas that may arise when there is confusion concerning roles within the setting in which the team operates. This problem can be equally complicated within the team itself if there is a lack of clarity on questions concerning the differentiation and integration of individual roles (Zander, Cohen, and Stotland, 1957; Mill, 1960). The differentiation of roles has been discussed elsewhere in the book, and we have highlighted the integration of roles through the case illustration with which we began the chapter. A few additional comments dealing with difficulties created when role problems are not resolved may be helpful, because the team's effectiveness depends to a great extent upon their resolution.

As we have stressed, change is constantly occurring in each of the professions involved in the diagnostic team, as well as in each specific team (Krugman et al., 1950). This leads to a constant need to redefine the role of each profession in relation to the others (Modlin and Faris, 1956). In this learning of roles, two opposite kinds of attitudes are often observed, with many gradations in between. On the one hand, the psychiatrist may be said to have the most important position on the team. On the other hand, under the guise of equality, any team member may be said to be qualified to do the job of any other team member, with or without the special training required. Equality, however, does not mean a blurring of roles. If everyone did the same thing and if each member were interchangeable with the other, no interdisciplinary team could exist and the opportunity of looking at the family from different perspectives would be lost. The problem of hierarchy, status, and interchangeability of roles does not even arise, however, if team functioning is properly understood. Instead of meaning that everybody does or could do each other's job, team functioning means that everyone plays an equally important role, in that each worker has an area that is essential to the team's success and, thus, one role is as important as any other (Allen, 1948). The question of which or who is more important is really a false issue. As the case of Mr. and Mrs. G. and Harold showed earlier, the psychiatrist and the psychologist can understand and work effectively with the child only in the light of the social worker's process with the parents, and, similarly, the social worker can work on the parents' role in the problem only if she is given a steady flow of information about the child.

An illustration of some of the difficulties that can arise in role differentiation occurred at the clinic during a regular training seminar on psychological testing attended by all disciplines. Again, the purpose of the seminar was not to make psychologists out of the other members but to familiarize them with the psychologists' role and the techniques used in fulfilling it. In this particular seminar, a senior psychologist would test a child currently undergoing evaluation in a one-way vision room. On one occasion, a child became extremely resistant, so the psychologist shifted to an interview approach designed to lay the foundation for a subsequent effort at testing. The psychiatric trainees, however, became highly incensed because they felt the psychologist was stepping out of his role and getting into their area. They then went to their psychiatric supervisor to complain that the psychologist had interfered with the role of the examining team psychiatrist. After talking with the psychologist, the supervising psychiatrist was able to see that the criticism was unjust; rather, the problem lay in the fact that psychiatric trainees held very stereotyped ideas as to the psychologist's function and the methods he should use in fulfilling this function. As a result, the supervising psychiatrist handled the problem in a conference with his trainees.

The senior psychologist in the M. case we discussed provided the correct approach to the dilemma arising from confusion over team roles. "The difficulty with the child in this case," he said, "is that he can't stick out the task of completing a test. The problem, then, is in not getting enough test samples; in fact, I would consider this problem even larger if I were an eager beaver who felt the tests had to be given fully or if I were test-centered and felt my job was to get a test response. Then, this type of case would be anxiety-arousing. However, I can deal with this kind of difficulty to the extent that I realize that I don't have to get a test response, that my job is to understand the child and what I use to achieve this appraisal is secondary. Of course, the more information I have, the more reliable it is, but without a full battery I can reach some conclusions anyway. Even the fact that I can or cannot test the boy is of significance itself." We can see, then, that the team needs to be flexible enough to allow each discipline to use the resources required to obtain an understanding of the child.

Other difficulties can arise from the attitude that a member of one discipline may have toward another (Lefton, Rettig, Dinitz, and Pasamanick, 1961). For instance, it is sometimes observed that the social worker tends to be used more readily as a scapegoat than other team members. Perhaps, among other factors, this is still a problem of status, related to the shorter period of initial training. An analysis of our conferences shows that everyone feels free to make suggestions to the social worker as to how to deal with parents, while team members (or supervisors from other disciplines)' seldom suggest what the psychologist or the psychiatrist should do in their processes with a child.

A problem sometimes occurs when the psychiatric trainees feel that the psychologist's methods are more scientific and, therefore, more valid than those of psychiatry, or that the psychologist's tests can reach a deeper level of understanding than the psychiatrist can achieve. In part, this problem may also be the result of a misconception common to trainees: namely, that the psychologist and psychiatrist must come up with the same picture of the child. Of course, this expectation is not valid; as we have stressed, the purpose in having the child seen by both psychiatrist and psychologist is to get pictures of the child from different points of view. Often, these pictures will be different, because the child may respond in one way to the psychologist's approach and in quite another way to that of the psychiatrist as we have seen. In order to avoid both overcritical attitudes and overvaluing attitudes, which may be especially damaging, Ruesch (1956) stresses the importance of double-group membership. By this he means working not only at tasks confined to the individual's professional group but at tasks in the interdisciplinary group as well. In this way, the individual is helped to keep his bearings and not be overwhelmed by other disciplines.

Another problem related to the differentiation of roles is the important question of what might be called talking outside one's own field. Can one discipline question another discipline? For example, can the social worker validly question the neurologist's findings, and vice versa? We believe they can and should, but in a particular way—that is, from their own frame of reference. For instance, in the first case illustration we discussed, the neurologist felt Harold's club foot had little influence on his present coordination difficulties, and from a strictly neurological-physical standpoint, this opinion could be correct. The social worker, however, could justifiably ask questions on the basis of the impact that such a defect would have upon the parents (and, in fact, we know they reacted to it by overindulging and overprotecting the boy, which could have delayed his practicing and learning motor skills). In this way, each team member absorbs, examines, reflects upon, and challenges information from the other members, but he does so from the framework of his own discipline.

Role Integration

The problem of integrating the various roles is as complex as differentiating them and, similarly, is sometimes not successfully resolved. As we tried to make clear, interdisciplinary team functioning requires integrating the findings of the various disciplines *throughout* the process as they emerge; in other words, the team cannot wait and put them together at the end. Our case illustration of Harold and his parents showed how the team members added to each other's understanding of their own findings, as well as to the total process, as the case developed. However, when such integration does not occur, serious errors may result.

If the team views the child from only one perspective without considering all the available evidence, this evidence can not be properly assessed and integrated. This also happens if some of the specialists on a case make separate reports without considering the findings of other team members. The sometimes prevalent notion that a more accurate examination will result if it is not "contaminated" by information from other disciplines is not wholly valid in diagnostic work. Each discipline may offer important questions that can be answered only by another; or the implications of certain data may not be clear until they are seen in relation to the rest of the information. Of course, many of the details and techniques that go into each specialist's process are of no particular interest or value to the other team members, who are interested primarily in the conclusions. For example, the social worker does not need to know how the psychologist goes about scoring the Rorschach, but he is interested in knowing what the psychologist interprets from his scoring. Each specialist, then, must distill and synthesize from his own process that which is useful to the other members' work.

LEADERSHIP

Problems of leadership have often given rise to much confusion in the interdisciplinary team. It is this confusion that we will try to clarify, rather than to deal much with leadership itself. In the first place, the problem is complicated by the fact that within the interdisciplinary team different levels of leadership exist, ranging from the chairman or consultant or director, as the case may be, to the supervisors and other senior members down to the members within the actual team itself—all of whom may, at one time or another, exert some amount of leadership during the process.

The issue of team leadership has become complicated by certain misconceptions about what it means to function as a team. Just as a problem about equality of team members may arise, so, too, a related confusion may occur over the question of leadership. Some erroneously believe that team functioning automatically means that everyone has an equal share in decision making and that no one individaul is more in charge than another or more competent to lead. Such a state of affairs, of course, would be chaos and is based on unsound assumptions. The opposite type of leadership—dictatorial decision making—is not useful in team functioning either. Leadership and authority are essential to a team, but the kind needed is quite different from that in which the leader does the thinking and the others carry it out (Brodey, 1961). If the leader runs the team in this fashion, they will be limited to what he sees, if the team rebels against such a leader, they will have to forego these insights.

Under any circumstances, the nature of the leadership will

have a vital influence on how the team will function. Problems will arise, for example, if the team leader favors one discipline over another; if he thinks only psychological tests are really valid, he will not "hear" the other findings, or if he believes the social work with the parents is not very important, he will underplay the social work role. If the leader is too restrictive, he will inhibit team spontaneity, but if he is too permissive, he will let the team drift. However, if he is too domineering, he will suppress or infantilize the team, but if he expects the members to function too independently, they will end up doing his work.

A strong leader can sometimes successfully rescue a process from failure, as illustrated by the following case. A recently widowed, very disturbed mother came for help for one of her young children, who was also seriously disturbed. Initially, she reacted to her interviews in the office by becoming increasingly disorganized. The team members and even some of the supervisors became concerned and felt the evaluation study would have to be terminated. The leader, however, suggested that the mother be seen in a less formal way—outside with her children playing around her, at the hospital cafeteria for coffee, and with both the psychiatrist and social worker present. Under these circumstances, the mother relaxed and became much better organized, so that the team was able to move ahead and help her in a significant way. In contrast, a weak leader would only have increased the team's dilemma, as in one case in which the leader withdrew from the outset and remained uninvolved and pessimistic.

Sometimes the leader has to choose a solution that will be unpopular; if he is insecure about going against the group or if the group's affection is too important to him, he may be unable to take the action that is needed for the best handling of the case. A strong difference of opinion puts both the leader and the group in a difficult position; if this occurs too often, the group might become too rebellious, possibly too resentful to function usefully. They might soon come to feel that it did not matter what they thought or recommended, since the leader would do as he pleased anyway. They might then cease to take responsibility for careful performance.

Not only the formally designated leader, but the senior

members and supervisors of the team can be of great help in leading, as we have illustrated earlier. Only a few brief comments can
be added here about such an extensive topic as supervision (Ekstein and Wallerstein, 1958; Fleming, 1953, 1966; Mathews and
Wineman, 1953). One of the many functions a supervisor of diagnostic work performs is to prevent the younger workers from reading too much into fragmentary or one-sided evidence. This is one
of the hazards of short-term diagnostic studies. Team members cannot wait for as much evidence to emerge as in a long-term therapeutic process, yet, on the other hand, they cannot act primarily on
the basis of speculation. Another problem the supervisor may have
to handle is the anxiety that a team member may feel when he cannot get information the other members would like him to provide.
He may feel that he is letting them down and is not doing his job
well. Here, again, his supervisor can help him get a more realistic
picture not only of what he is expected to do in general but what
he can do in a particular case. Although team functioning will tend
to increase the quality of individual performance because each
member feels a responsibility toward his teammates, it can also create unnecessary anxiety. Such anxiety occurs either because the individual has unrealistically high expectations of what he should be
able to provide or feels pressed to provide more than is actually
possible. Sometimes another member creates this feeling because of
difficulties in his own process, which he hopes someone else will
solve in his work.

Supervisors must also be alert to the lack of awareness that
new members may have of the total process, along with their resistance to thinking about and taking responsibility for this totality.
New members, who are primarily involved with their own roles,
may think of the case only sectionally and want to leave the integration up to someone else. They hope someone else will do it for
them or may even believe someone else is supposed to do it for
them—the supervisor, the conference chairman, or another team
member. In the final analysis, the team must move toward an integration, a synthesis of all the contributions, with each profession
taking responsibility for its own area and the decisions made within
it. Despite the fact that each team member is somewhat self-in-

volved in the beginning, he does gradually become open to other factors and is able to move toward an integrated view of the whole case.

Sometimes, of course, the senior team members may be less helpful than they should be. A situation familiar to all is the one in which the senior people dominate the meetings and do not give the junior members an opportunity to express their observations and thoughts. It is important to create an atmosphere in which each member, new or old, feels that his ideas are listened to with respect, even though everyone may not agree with them. This receptive climate is a vital aspect of the trainee's experience; it contributes to his growth and will be missed if easy interchange becomes difficult or impossible. If the new member is afraid his contributions are either unwanted or subject to unfair criticism, he will not feel free to make them. Of course, much also depends on the skill, experience, and maturity of the new members; some will be ready to think along with the senior people at a higher level of integration, while others will not. But all members at whatever level should give fair consideration to ideas of other members of the team.

Another problem sometimes observed in teamwork is competition among the senior people. They may engage in intellectual pyrotechnics with each other, while the real work purpose of the conference is lost. Perhaps a supervisor may relate to those he supervises as a jealous parent and be reluctant to allow them to learn from contacts with other workers and other disciplines. Still another problem may come from a senior member's knowingly or unknowingly providing substitute supervision for a trainee in another discipline. For example, if a psychiatrist is flattered by the attentions of a social work trainee who claims he knows more or handles something better than his own supervisor, the psychiatrist may initiate a power struggle by acting as an advisor to the trainee. For example, the psychologist or social worker may not only have a supervisor from his own discipline but one from psychiatry because of the medical responsibility involved in a case (Siporin and Boshes, 1957). A worker may also circumvent the proper channel of supervision, by trying to get supervision from the team as a whole or from a specific team member. Another possible variation results when a worker does not deal directly with his fellow team member but instead, for one reason or another, attempts to go directly to a team member's supervisor for information. For instance, in a discussion seminar for new workers at the clinic, a psychology trainee recalled his anger toward one of the social workers because in his first several cases with her, she constantly went to his supervisor for information instead of coming to him. His reaction was "If that's the way you want it, I won't see you at all." From the seminar it emerged that this particular social worker felt she was not getting enough help in her own supervision, and as a result—though she was unaware of the connection at the time—she did not trust the psychology trainee's supervision either. This situation again highlights how problems in one discipline can create difficulties in working with other disciplines as well.

Differences of opinion about a case are bound to occur among the supervisors as well as among the more junior team members. Disagreement, of course, is not necessarily bad. There is a need to keep an open mind to the possible range of facts and contributions from various specialties. However, the reasons for these differences of opinion must be explored. Too, respect for such differences will be much more possible when good will and empathy exist among the team members for each other. Empathy itself does not imply agreement but means, instead, a recognition of the other persons' contributions. When differences of opinion do arise in the team they should be on the basis of variations in data or different, but rational, interpretations of the evidence—certainly not on disagreement rooted in emotional conflict. Differences have to be presented to the family in the same objective way; family members should not be told that there is *conflict* about certain issues, but that some questions cannot be fully resolved or finally answered at this point.

Honest differences of interpretation are healthful for the process and can contribute to a necessary open-mindedness and lack of dogmatism on the part of the team. On the other hand, differences of viewpoint and philosophies that are too extreme can lead to such complications as power struggles and "in" and "out" groups and, as a result, can have a detrimental effect on the integration of the team and, ultimately, on the effectiveness of the work done with the family. For example, in the W. case, the senior psychiatrist and senior psychologist did not work together smoothly because of an underlying conflict not related to the task at hand. At the final conference, the team psychiatrist said at one point, "I keep feeling something is missing here and I can't quite handle it. Something is floating around that I can't grasp." We believe that what was floating around beyond his grasp was the conflict between the senior psychiatrist and the supervising psychologist. The other team members were, of course, not directly aware of the difficulty, which the senior psychologist brought only indirectly into the picture. Apparently, he wished to show that the senior psychiatrist was in error, and, as a result, displaced to the team situation the disagreement the two of them were having in an unrelated situation. The case ended with a general feeling of dissatisfaction on everyone's part. Although this might have been the result anyway because of the complexity of the case, the chance for success would have been better if the junior team members had not had to work with this difficult family when their own family was divided.

The third level of leadership in the interdisciplinary team is leadership among the actual team members themselves. Of course, the medical responsibility in a psychiatric setting carries with it a certain requirement in leadership that will naturally fall to the medical member of the team. In addition to this aspect, however, a variety of other factors complicate and influence the question of leadership, including the skill and experience of the individual members, personality factors such as the degree of initiative and ambition to lead, and team culture patterns (for example, "who gets listened to most by whom"). To lead requires a certain level of confidence based on training and experience, although all the team members are free to lead according to the case needs. Distrust of a teammate's leadership and competitiveness of one member that prevents the proper leadership of another member are only two of the many covert factors that can interrupt the proper interchange of leadership roles required in team functioning.

In a well-balanced and smoothly working team, the crucial factor that determines which team member leads at any particular

point is what is taking place at that moment in the process. Sometimes, the social worker will in a sense have the more dominant
role; at another time, it may be, for example, the neurologist or
the psychologist. This changing pattern was observed in the G. case.
At one point the information the psychiatrist supplied about the
possibility of the child's being brain-damaged was significant in fur-
thering understanding, and, for the time being, he was the leader;
on another occasion, the focus and leadership shifted to the social
worker's problems with the parents; and later still, the psychologist
became the leader when the child's responses to the CAT stories
were the most helpful in understanding the case at that moment.
When there are comfortable relationships among the team members, then, variation in leadership adapted to the case needs, and
not to some internal needs, will occur.

INTRATEAM COMMUNICATION

Much of what we have previously discussed relates to the
question of intrateam communication (Moriarty, 1961). In the interdisciplinary process itself, there are inherent problems of communication (Cunningham, 1952), which are of two general types.
The first concerns the fact that communication must go on between special groups, each with its own particular training and experience and, to some extent, with its own special language. The
second concerns problems common to any group, such as over-
crowded schedules, poor geographical arrangements, too rigid hierarchies, intrateam conflicts, and divisive personality characteristics,
perhaps an overbearing attitude toward others or a tendency to se-
clusiveness and a preference for working alone.

In the first type, communication among the different fields
becomes difficult when each specialty, in many instances, uses the
same words but with different meanings for different disciplines
(Cunningham, 1952). The reverse of this occurs when the disciplines have differing technical terms for the same thing. Part of
the process of group development involves becoming aware of and
then resolving some of these language difficulties. Eventually, to
some extent, a common language is developed, and understanding
is achieved at least about those terms which are not used in com-

mon. A related problem is the too frequent use of jargon, a practice which is all too often followed by new and old members alike (Deveraux, 1950). This can serve a number of purposes: it may be used to hide a lack of knowledge, to try to impress a colleague, or, probably most frequently, to avoid having to make the effort of really thinking something through so that it can be simply and clearly expressed.

In the second type of problem in team communication—encompassing difficulties common to any group—the main factor is, of course, the complexity of the operation in which a great number and variety of people are involved in varying ways and degrees (Knoff, Mabry, and Stainbrook, 1958). Too often because of the pressure of time, and the geographical distance between some of the team members, as well as because of other factors, intrateam contact may have a hurried, hit-or-miss quality. Information is shared on the run without allowing sufficient time for a careful weighing and discussion of its implications. While much can be said for spontaneity, there can be serious disadvantages to this when important information must be exchanged, for example, over coffee; distractions usually mark such an informal meeting, data and impressions may be tossed out but not always listened to carefully or considered reflectively.

The question of the optimum number of people to have in the group is also an important one from the viewpoint of communication. In certain respects, adding even more people to the regular team membership, perhaps from such disciplines as pediatrics or sociology, might be fruitful, but, on the other hand, the addition might make the team too unwieldy and thus defeat the purpose. In a smaller group, there is a greater chance for individual contributions, although the range of ideas and knowledge that will be brought to bear on the case will be narrower. Also, in a small group, if conflicts occur among the members, they may be more intensely felt and expressed. The fewer the members, the more obvious each person's individual idiosyncrasies will be. A small group also makes greater demands for performance and participation by each member. However, the more familiar the members are with each other—unless there is conflict—the more free they will be in their communication with each other and the more time they will have for such expression. When a number of people besides the actual team members are present for teaching or other purposes, the nonmembers may dominate the discussion or bring up issues that are not of immediate, practical relevance for the team; as a result, the team members may leave the conference in frustration because their needs have not been met. Again, a balance must be found between teaching needs and service needs.

At times, too much communication may take place either between individual members or at group meetings, with the participants involving themselves in discussions that avoid the central problem and become enmeshed in side issues or that degenerate into competitive struggles or social interchanges. In the L. case, for instance, the team psychologist and the team psychiatrist, who were personal friends, met frequently because they enjoyed visiting with each other, rather than because they wished to discuss the specific needs of the case. In the W. case, team communication was hampered by the struggle going on between the senior psychologist and the senior psychiatrist; in fact, the senior psychologist did not even hear certain material because of this struggle.

Another problem arises when team members listen to each other's points of view overreceptively. This situation may occur if they are already anxious about their own process and have hopes that other data will solve their problems for them. Thus, the team member having difficulty with his own process is more susceptible to what he hears because he needs it so much. It is also necessary to learn *what* is useful to share from one's own discipline and *when* it is helpful to share it. If the quality of communication and the reception by the members are good, findings do not take too long to communicate. Young workers, however, sometimes lack sufficient breadth of knowledge to make a clear and concise presentation possible.

A group discussion on communication dealt with some of the above issues during a training seminar held for new team members. It emerged that the psychiatrists and the psychologists felt the social workers became too involved with the material about the child to give close attention to information on the parents. The social workers all insisted that they were eager to hear as soon as possible about the child, but the psychiatrists were divided in their feelings as to their need to hear immediately about the parents. Some of the social workers also believed that it was important for them, after the first contact with the parents, to see the psychiatrist, but less important to see the psychologist. One of the psychologists pointed out that if the other members seemed interested in his findings, he was pleased, but if not, he felt his work was being shrugged off as unimportant. (To some extent this reaction could reflect an individual problem; if a team member is doubtful about his worth and value—as a new member often is—he would be more sensitive in this way.)

Another point brought out in this meeting was that sometimes in the initial stage of the case process beginning members were so anxious about their work that in their communications they contributed anxiety rather than constructive information helpful to the other team members. A psychology trainee observed that he did not feel particularly willing to communicate when he was having difficulty in testing a child and also admitted that he found himself rather pleased if the psychiatrist was having difficulty too. This attitude, however, made trouble in the specific case from which he was generalizing, because in the preconference at which these two members shared their anxiety about their patient, the social worker began to become anxious, too.

Some of the trainees in this seminar complained about the lack of direction on what and when to communicate, even though they also recognized that this knowledge is gradually learned. The problem of presenting information in too much detail was also brought up, and, again, several of the social workers reported that they shared little information about the parents because they felt that no one was very much interested in it. Significantly, the director had expressed to an observer at about the time of the seminar that social work at the clinic seemed almost a private practice, because details of the actual process between parents and social workers were never communicated in the conferences, or even put in the final case write-up. He felt that, for some reason, the social workers did not want to share this information. However, it now became apparent from this seminar discussion that the social workers felt they should limit their observations because nobody seemed to be interested in hearing about them.

Obviously, of the many ways in which team difficulties can be handled, the most important is by prevention (Ness, 1954). Ideally, then, an administrative setup that encourages and facilitates good team functioning is necessary to provide well-planned physical facilities and a well-qualified staff of adequate size, as well as to see that relationships with other groups are harmoniously integrated with the outpatient group. Time must be provided to examine, reflect, and communicate properly, along with the channels essential for these activities. Provisions must also be made for good leadership and good supervision, which will not only give support, but will encourage growth, inspire enthusiasm, and facilitate research. Care must go into selecting personnel who are not only varied enough in both training and interests to prevent slipping into a comfortable but rigid routine, but who are flexible and mature enough to work well with others in a shared undertaking. Assigning team members varied responsibilities has distinct advantages, too, since one of the beneficial results is cross-fertilization. Members of each discipline should also have their own as well as interdisciplinary meetings, their own supervision, and their own areas of responsibility—all of which are equally valued by the administration.

But in spite of the best efforts along these lines, difficulties will inevitably arise from time to time. We have stressed that intrateam relationships are not constant and unchanging. They are constantly shifting and altering and are accepted, challenged, weakened, and strengthened by the activities and relationships of the members. Some problems require administrative solutions, ranging from instituting a different time structure to shifting personnel or making changes in members' responsibilities. Sometimes it is helpful to have those who are at odds over one issue work on something else on which they can agree. As a result, they may be able to see the viewpoints they have in common and thus be able to solve the previous problem. This approach does not always work, however, because the other problem may carry over to the new situation, as indicated in the W. case, in which we pointed out that the conflict between the supervisors carried over to the diagnostic area.

Some problems are resolved without the awareness of the individuals involved. Such a resolution comes about through working together and from the informal education that team members receive in every team meeting and in every interaction with each other. Some education may take place more formally through supervision and through other planned educational efforts. In our setting we have found it useful to have training seminars such as the ones we discussed earlier, in which the focus is upon the various aspects of outpatient teamwork, which is outside the usual areas covered in supervision.

Attempts at improvement based on education or on better communication will be of no avail if more basic difficulties sabotage these measures. For example, the frequent complaint of inadequate communication is a familiar one, usually referring to the feeling of a lack of flow of information from the top down in the hierarchy or horizontally, so to speak, between disciplines, rather than from the bottom up. While such complaints are often justified, the common tendency, nevertheless, is for people to project their own inner conflicts onto the structure around them; if these conflicts, then, are the underlying problem, the attempt to solve it by increased communication, better job definitions, or organizational changes will fail (Cohen, 1956).

As far as the individual's problems are concerned, some can be handled merely by further training and experience (Connery, 1951), some can only be resolved through psychotherapy, and some cannot be handled at all since some people, for one reason or another, never really function satisfactorily in a team. The latter may belong to that group of individuals who do their best work on their own; when for some reason such individuals are put in the position of having to work with a group, the results are likely to be unhappy for everyone concerned.

Finally, in considering what to do about individual problems, we must include a word of warning against thinking of the interdisciplinary team as a therapeutic group—a warning against the common tendency of wanting to solve individual problems through having teammates interpret them. The belief is sometimes erroneously held that in good teamwork all feelings and problems should be freely expressed by everybody. This is somehow taken to mean that the group is then really working together, and, thus, all difficulties will somehow be magically resolved. While free expression may help in certain situations, it by no means always does; in fact, such a practice can easily get out of hand, be used aggressively by various individuals, and do far more harm than good. Also, members have different tolerances for open expression of feelings and different degrees of flexibility in being able to deal with them. It is not the group's concern to diagnose why various members feel or react the way they do. Actually, nothing is more irritating than to have someone on the team attempt to "interpret" why one is doing thus or so. Rarely do such maneuvers solve anything, and very often they lead to further conflict.

Perhaps when the above occurs, listening—true listening—has stopped, and the major purpose of the study has become blurred. In the final analysis, as stated earlier, the team must move toward an integration, a synthesis of all of the contributions, with each member taking responsibility for his own area and the decisions within it. Ideally, the design of such a synthesis should give a coherent and comprehensive understanding of the child and his family so that the next steps—what should be done, and what can be done—are sound and hopeful. This goal is more near achievement when each team member has listened carefully, not only to the child and to his parents, not only to his own thoughts and emotions, but to those of his colleagues as well. It is a truism that when each team member has felt understood and has felt growth and gain in knowledge and empathy, the family members experience this also and report gain and growth in their capacity to face the future. This is the ultimate goal and an essential step in the treatment to follow.

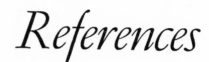

References

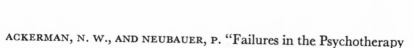

ACKERMAN, N. W., AND NEUBAUER, P. "Failures in the Psychotherapy of Children." In P. H. Hoch (Ed.), *Failures in Psychiatric Treatment*. New York: Grune and Stratton, 1948.

ALLEN, F. H. "Psychiatry and Social Work in Cooperation." *American Journal of Psychiatry*, 1948, *104*, 554–557.

ALLEN, F. H. *Psychotherapy with Children*. New York: Norton, 1942.

American Psychiatric Association. *Career Training in Child Psychiatry*. Washington, D.C.: American Psychiatric Association, 1964.

BARBARA, D. A. (Ed.) *Psychological and Psychiatric Aspects of Speech and Hearing*. Springfield, Ill.: Thomas, 1960.

279

BENDA, C. E. *Developmental Disorders of Mentation and Cerebral Palsies.* New York: Grune and Stratton, 1952.

BLOS, P. *On Adolescence.* New York: Free Press, 1962.

BORNSTEIN, B. "Emotional Barriers in the Understanding and Treatment of Young Children." *American Journal of Orthopsychiatry,* 1948, *18,* 691–697.

BORNSTEIN, B. "On Latency." *Psychoanalytic Study of the Child,* 1951, *6,* 279–285.

BRENNER, C. *An Elementary Textbook of Psychoanalysis.* New York: International Universities Press, 1955.

BRODEY, M. W. "The Psychiatric Case Conference." *Psychiatry,* 1961, *24,* 361–366.

BRODEY, M. W., AND HAYDEN, M. "Intrateam Reactions: Their Relation to the Conflicts of the Family in Treatment." *American Journal of Orthopsychiatry,* 1957, *27,* 349–355.

BRODNITZ, F. S. *Vocal Rehabilitation.* Rochester, Minn.: Whiting Press, 1959.

BUXBAUM, E. "A Contribution to the Psychoanalytic Knowledge of the Latency Period." *American Journal of Orthopsychiatry,* 1951, *21,* 182–198.

CAUDILL, W. A. *The Psychiatric Hospital as a Small Society.* Cambridge: Harvard University Press, 1958.

CHESS, S. *Introduction to Child Psychiatry.* New York: Grune and Stratton, 1959.

COHEN, I. H. Quoted in "Staff Discomforts and the Social Organization of a Mental Hospital" by Otto Pollak. *Psychiatry,* 1956, *19,* 314.

CONNERY, M. F. "Problems in Teaching the Team Concept." *Journal of Psychiatric Social Work,* 1951, *21,* 81–89.

CRITCHLEY, M. *Developmental Dyslexia.* Springfield, Ill.: Thomas, 1964.

CRUTCHER, R. "Child Psychiatry: A History of Its Development." *Psychiatry,* 1943, *6,* 191–201.

CUNNINGHAM, J. M. "Problems of Communication in Scientific and Professional Disciplines." *American Journal of Orthopsychiatry,* 1952, *22,* 445–456.

Dartmouth Conference. *Education for Psychiatric Social Work.* New York: American Association for Psychiatric Social Workers, 1950.

DAVIS, H. (Ed.) *Hearing and Deafness.* New York: Holt, 1960.

DEUTSCH, H. *The Psychology of Women: A Psychoanalytic Interpretation,* two volumes. New York: Grune and Stratton, 1944–1945.

DEVEREUX, G. "Some Unconscious Determinants of the Use of Technical Terms in Psychoanalytic Writing." *Bulletin of the Menninger Clinic,* 1950, *14,* 202–206.

DITTES, J. E., AND KELLEY, H. H. "Effects of Different Conditions of Acceptance upon Conformity to Group Norms." *Journal of Abnormal and Social Psychology,* 1956, *53,* 100–107.

EIDUSON, B. T. *Psychiatric Case History Event System Transcription Procedures with Lexicons.* Los Angeles: Reiss-Davis Child Study Center, 1966.

EISENSON, J. *Stuttering: A Symposium.* New York: Harper, 1958.

EKSTEIN, R., AND WALLERSTEIN, R. S. *The Teaching and Learning of Psychotherapy.* New York: Basic Books, 1958.

ENGLISH, O. S., AND PEARSON, G. H. J. *Common Neuroses of Children and Adults.* New York: Norton, 1937.

ENGLISH, O. S., AND PEARSON, G. H. J. *Emotional Problems of Living.* (2nd ed.) New York: Norton, 1955.

ERIKSON, E. H. *Childhood and Society.* (2nd ed.) New York: Norton, 1963.

ERIKSON, E. H. "Growth and Crises of the Healthy Personality." *Psychological Issues,* 1959, *1,* 50–100.

ERIKSON, E. H. "The Problem of Ego Identity." *Journal of the American Psychoanalytic Association,* 1956, *4,* 56–121.

ESCALONA, S. "Emotional Development in the First Year of Life." In M. J. E. Senn (Ed.), *Problems of Infancy and Childhood.* New York: Josiah Macy, Jr., Foundation, 1953.

FINCH, S. M. *Fundamentals of Child Psychiatry.* New York: Norton, 1960.

FLEMING, J. "The Role of Supervision in Psychiatric Training." *Bulletin of the Menninger Clinic,* 1953, *17,* 157–169.

FLEMING, J., AND BENEDEK, T. F. *Psychoanalytic Supervision.* New York: Grune and Stratton, 1966.

FORD, F. R. *Diseases of the Nervous System in Infancy, Childhood and Adolescence.* (5th ed.) Springfield, Ill.: Thomas, 1966.

FRANK, L. K. "Play in Personality Development." *American Journal of Orthopsychiatry,* 1955, *25,* 576–590.

FREUD, A. "Indications for Child Anaylsis." *Psychoanalytic Study of the Child,* 1945, *1,* 127–149.

FREUD, A. *The Psycho-Analytical Treatment of Children.* London: Imago, 1946.

FRIEND, M. R. "An Evaluation from the Psychiatric Point of View." In O. Pollak et al. (Eds.), *Social Science and Psychotherapy for Children.* New York: Russell Sage Foundation, 1952.

GARDNER, G. E. "Clinical Research in a Child Psychiatry Setting." *American Journal of Orthopsychiatry,* 1956, *26,* 330–339.

Group for the Advancement of Psychiatry, Committee on Child Psychiatry. *Basic Concepts in Child Psychiatry* (GAP Report No. 12). New York: Group for the Advancement of Psychiatry, 1950.

Group for the Advancement of Psychiatry, Committee on Child Psychiatry. *The Diagnostic Process in Child Psychiatry* (GAP Report No. 38). New York: Group for the Advancement of Psychiatry, 1957.

HALPERN, F. "The Individual Psychological Examination." In M. G. Gottsegen and G. B. Gottsegen (Eds.), *Professional School Psychology.* New York: Grune and Stratton, 1960.

HARRISON, S. I., AND CAREK, D. J. *A Guide to Psychotherapy.* Boston: Little, Brown, 1966.

HARTMANN, H. *Ego Psychology and the Problem of Adaptation.* New York: International Universities Press, 1958.

HEALY, W. *The Individual Delinquent.* Boston: Little, Brown, 1915.

HSIA, D. Y. *Inborn Errors of Metabolism.* (2nd ed.) Chicago: Year Book Medical Publishers, 1966.

JERGER, J. F. (Ed.) *Modern Developments in Audiology.* New York: Academic Press, 1963.

JOSSELYN, I. M. *The Adolescent and His World.* New York: Family Service Association of America, 1952.

KANNER, L. *Child Psychiatry.* (3rd ed.) Springfield, Ill.: Thomas, 1957.

KANNER, L. "Child Psychiatry: Retrospect and Prospect." *American Journal of Psychiatry,* 1960, *117,* 15–22.

KESSLER, J. W. *Psychopathology of Childhood.* Englewood Cliffs, N.J.: Prentice-Hall, 1966.

KLEIN, M. "Our Adult World and Its Roots in Infancy." *Human Relations,* 1959, *12,* 291–303.

KNOFF, W. F., MABRY, J. H., AND STAINBROOK, E. J. "Social Structure and Verbal Participation in the Psychiatric Case Conference." In P. H. Hoch and J. Zubin (Eds.), *Psychopathology of Communication.* New York: Grune and Stratton, 1958.

KRUGMAN, M., et al. "A Study of Current Trends in the Use and Coordination of Professional Services of Psychiatrists, Psychologists and Social Workers in Mental Hygiene Clinics and Other Psychiatric Agencies and Institutions." *American Journal of Orthopsychiatry,* 1950, *20,* 1–62.

LABARRE, M. "Dynamic Factors in Psychiatric Team Collaboration." *British Journal of Medical Psychology,* 1960, *33,* 53–60.

LEFTON, M., RETTIG, S., DINITZ, S., AND PASAMANICK, B. "Status Perceptions of Psychiatric Social Workers and Their Implications for Work Satisfaction." *American Journal of Orthopsychiatry,* 1961, *31,* 102–110.

LEVINE, M. "Principles of Psychiatric Treatment." In F. Alexander (Ed.), *Dynamic Psychiatry.* Chicago: University of Chicago Press, 1952.

LEVY, D. M. "A Method of Integrating Physical and Psychiatric Examination." *American Journal of Psychiatry,* 1929, *9,* 121–194.

LICHTENBERG, P. "Reactions to Success and Failure During Individual and Cooperative Effort." *Journal of Social Psychology,* 1957, *46,* 31–34.

LOWENFIELD, M., AND MABERLY, A. D. "Discussion on Value of Play Therapy in Child Psychiatry." *Proceedings of the Royal Society of Medicine,* 1946, *39,* 439–443.

MARKS, P. A. "An Assessment of the Diagnostic Process in a Child Guidance Setting." *Psychological Monographs,* 1961, *75*(3).

MATTHEWS, W. M., AND WINEMAN, D. "Supervision of Clinical Diagnostic Work." *American Journal of Orthopsychiatry,* 1953, *23,* 301–306.

MENNINGER, K. A. *A Manual for Psychiatric Case Study.* (2nd ed.) New York: Grune and Stratton, 1962.

MEYERS, H. L. "The Therapeutic Function of the Evaluation Process." *Bulletin of the Menninger Clinic,* 1956, *20,* 9–19.

MILL, C. R. "Interprofessional Awareness of Roles." *Journal of Clinical Psychology,* 1960, *16,* 411–413.

MODLIN, H. C., AND FARIS, M. "Follow-up Study of Psychiatric Team Functioning." *Bulletin of the Menninger Clinic,* 1954, *18,* 242–251.

MODLIN, H. C., AND FARIS, M. "Group Adaptation and Integration in Psychiatric Team Practice." *Psychiatry,* 1956, *19,* 97–103.

MODLIN, H. C., GARDNER, R. W., AND FARIS, M. "Implications of a Therapeutic Process in Evaluations by Psychiatric Teams." *American Journal of Orthopsychiatry,* 1958, *28,* 647–655.

MORIARTY, J. D. "Problems in Communication for the Psychiatrist." *Diseases of the Nervous System,* 1961, *22,* 109–113.

MYKLEBUST, H. R. *Auditory Disorders in Children.* New York: Grune and Stratton, 1954.

NESS, C. M. "The Influence of Administration upon Interprofessional Harmony." *Journal of Psychiatric Social Work,* 1954, *24,* 29–30.

PAINE, R. S., AND OPPÉ, T. E. *Neurological Examination of Children.* London: Heinemann, 1966.

PEARSON, G. H. J. *Emotional Disorders of Children.* New York: Norton, 1949.

PELLER, L. E. "Libidinal Phases, Ego Development and Play." *Psychoanalytic Study of the Child,* 1954, *9,* 178–198.

PERLMAN, H. H. "Intake and Some Role Considerations." *Social Casework,* 1960, *41,* 171–177.

PIAGET, J. *Play, Dreams, and Imitation.* New York: Norton, 1951.

POLLAK, O., et al. (Eds.) *Social Science and Psychotherapy for Children.* New York: Russell Sage Foundation, 1952.

RAINES, G. N., AND ROHERER, J. H. "The Operational Matrix of Psychiatric Practice: Variability in Psychiatric Impressions and the Projection Hypothesis." *American Journal of Psychiatry,* 1960, *117,* 133–139.

RANK, B., AND MACNAUGHTON, D. "A Clinical Contribution to Early Ego Development." *Psychoanalytic Study of the Child,* 1950, *5,* 53–65.

RETTIG, S., JACOBSON, F. N., AND PASAMANICK, B. "The Motivational Pattern of the Mental Health Professional." In B. Pasamanick and P. H. Knapp (Eds.), *Social Aspects of Psychiatry* (Psychiatric Research Reports #10). Washington, D.C.: American Psychiatric Association, 1958.

ROSS, A. O. *The Practice of Clinical Child Psychology.* New York: Grune and Stratton, 1959.

ROUSEY, C. L., AND MORIARTY, A. E. *Diagnostic Implications of Speech Sounds.* Springfield, Ill.: Thomas, 1965.

RUESCH, J. *Nonverbal Communication.* Berkeley: University of California Press, 1956.

SCOTT, W. C. M. "Differences Between the Playroom Used in Child Psychiatric Treatment and in Child Analysis." *Canadian Psychiatric Association Journal,* 1961, *6,* 281–285.

SHAPIRO, M. I. "Psychiatric Examination of the Child." *Mental Hygiene,* 1959, *43,* 32–39.

SIPORIN, M., AND BOSHES, B. "Current Aspects of Psychiatric Social Work Collaboration." *Diseases of the Nervous System,* 1957, *18,* 169–175.

STOTLAND, E. *The Psychology of Hope.* San Francisco: Jossey-Bass, 1969.

SULLIVAN, H. S. *The Psychiatric Interview.* New York: Norton, 1954.

TALLENT, N. *Clinical Psychological Consultation: A Rationale and Guide to Team Practice.* Englewood Cliffs, N.J.: Prentice-Hall, 1963.

TALLENT, N., AND REISS, W. J. "Multidisciplinary Views on the Preparation of Written Clinical Psychological Reports." *Journal of Clinical Psychology,* 1959, *15,* 444–446.

TEMPLIN, M. C. *Certain Language Skills in Children.* Minneapolis: University of Minnesota Press, 1957.

THELEN, H. A. *Dynamics of Groups at Work.* Chicago: University of Chicago Press, 1956.

TRAVIS, L. E. (Ed.) *Handbook of Speech Pathology.* New York: Appleton-Century-Crofts, 1957.

TUDDENHAM, R. D. "The Influence of a Distorted Group Norm upon Individual Judgment." *Journal of Psychology,* 1958, *46,* 227–241.

WAELDER, R. *Basic Theory of Psychoanalysis.* New York: International Universities Press, 1960.

WEINGARTEN, E. M. "A Study of Selective Perception in Clinical Judgment." *Journal of Personality,* 1949, *17,* 369–406.

WHITMAN, R. M. "The Rating and Group Dynamics of the Psychiatric Staff Conference." *Psychiatry,* 1956, *19,* 333–340.

WIENER, D. N., AND RATHS, O. N. "Contributions of the Mental Hygiene Clinic Team to Clinic Decisions." *American Journal of Orthopsychiatry,* 1959, *29,* 350–356.

YARROW, M. R., CAMPBELL, J. D., AND BURTON, R. V. *Child Rearing: An Inquiry into Research and Methods.* San Francisco: Jossey-Bass, 1968.

ZANDER, A., COHEN, A. R., AND STOTLAND, E. *Role Relations in the Mental Health Professions.* Ann Arbor: University of Michigan, Research Center for Group Dynamics, Institute for Social Research, 1957.

ZANDER, A., STOTLAND, E., AND WOLFE, D. "Unity of Group, Identi-

fication with Group, and Self-Esteem of Members."
Journal of Personality, 1960, *28,* 463–478.

ZILLER, R. C., AND BEHRINGER, R. D. "Assimilation of the Knowledgeable Newcomer Under Conditions of Group Success and Failure." *Journal of Abnormal and Social Psychology,* 1960, *60,* 288–291.

ZILLER, R. C., BEHRINGER, R. D., AND JANSEN, M. J. "The Newcomer in Open and Closed Groups." *Journal of Applied Psychology,* 1961, *45,* 55–58.

Index